Advances in Mental Health and Addiction

Series Editor
Masood Zangeneh, Richmond Hill, ON, Canada

Over the past several decades we have witnessed dramatic shifts in prevailing approaches to mental health and addiction. Significant scientific achievements have led to novel treatment options that impacted the experiences of individuals with mental disorders. In recent years, new perspectives have begun to influence the way we address mental health and substance dependencies, resulting in a greater emphasis on mental health promotion and prevention strategies. Despite these progressions, mental health care systems too often remain stagnant, fragmented, and peripheral.

Catherine Comiskey

Addiction Research and Evaluation

Addressing Key Challenges for Policy and Practice

Springer

Catherine Comiskey
Trinity College Dublin
The University of Dublin
Dublin, Ireland

ISSN 2570-3390 ISSN 2570-3404 (electronic)
Advances in Mental Health and Addiction
ISBN 978-3-031-65916-4 ISBN 978-3-031-65917-1 (eBook)
https://doi.org/10.1007/978-3-031-65917-1

This Springer imprint is published by the registered company Springer Nature Switzerland AG
The registered company address is: Gewerbestrasse 11, 6330 Cham, Switzerland

To my husband Peter Carroll and our four adult children, Seán, Shannon, Julia, and Molly, for their endless love, companionship, encouragement, and support. To my parents, Vera and Christy Comiskey for the education, values and love of learning that they gave my siblings, Paul, Geraldine, Anthony, Leslie, and I. Thank you all, you know I love you.

Series Editor's Preface

Addiction Research and Evaluation: Addressing Key Challenges for Policy and Practice aims to bridge the gap between research and practice in the field of addiction. Authored by Prof. Catherine Comiskey, this book offers a comprehensive guide for practitioners, scientists, and policymakers seeking to enhance their understanding and application of effective methodologies in addiction research and evaluation.

The complexities of addiction and the myriad of factors influencing it demand rigorous, evidence-based approaches. This book provides a step-by-step guide to robust methodologies and illustrative case studies that exemplify best practices in the field. By doing so, it aims to improve knowledge transfer and service delivery, ensuring that research findings are effectively translated into practical applications that can inform policy and improve outcomes for individuals affected by addiction.

Drawing from Prof. Comiskey's extensive experience and expertise, this book serves as an invaluable resource for those involved in addiction research, treatment, and policy-making. It addresses the key challenges faced by the field and offers practical solutions to overcome them, fostering a collaborative approach to addressing the complex issue of addiction.

I hope that this book will inspire and equip readers with the tools and insights needed to make meaningful contributions to the field of addiction research and evaluation. Together, we can work toward more effective and compassionate responses to addiction, ultimately improving the lives of those affected by this pervasive issue.

Competing Interests This author declares no competing interests.

Ethics Approval This manuscript reports on methodologies and secondary previously published studies. These previously published studies obtained informed consent from participants.

Richmond, ON, Canada Masood Zangeneh

Acknowledgments

I would like to acknowledge each of the persons who use substances and who gave of their time to my research over the years. You are the bravest, strongest, most inspiring people I know. Your courage continues to humble and inspire me to use the education I have been fortunate to receive to do impactful research and to share my findings and knowledge with those in a position to make a difference.

A special thank you to Dr. Elizabeth McCarthy who helped me with the referencing.

Finally, I would like to acknowledge each of my past and current doctoral candidates. Thank you all for your giving and receiving of support and for your sharing of learning with me, I continue to learn so much from you: Dr. Yoon Choi; Dr. Gloria Crispino; Dr. Éimear Smith; Dr. Emma White; Dr. Julian Pugh; Dr. Orla Dempsey; Dr. Katy Tobin; Dr. Anne Snel; Dr. Mary Quirke; Dr. Ciara Wynne; Dr. Mary O'Rourke; Dr. Catherine Walden; Dr. Eleanor Hollywood; Dr. Karin O'Sullivan; Dr. Emma Murphy; Dr. Aidan Hanaway; Dr. Prakashini (Sonam) Banka; Dr. Anne Marie Carew; Dr. Michelle Byrne; Dr. Jenny Gordon; Dr. Debra O'Neill; Dr. Karen Galligan; Dr. Dave McDonagh; Dr. Marie Hyland; Dr. Kristine Nicki Annunziata; Niall Breslin; Sarah Jackson; Sadie Lavell Cafferkey; Muluken Basa; Philip James; Gráinne Clarke; and Louise McCullough.

About the Book

According to the United Nations Office of Drugs and Crime around 284 million people aged between 15 and 64 years used drugs in the year 2020. While numbers are estimated at a global level there remains little evidence for practitioners and policy makers on key questions at local level.

Questions include the challenging topics of providing safe injecting spaces and drug consumption rooms. As populations age in some regions, questions arise on the nature of substance use among older people. Countries with younger populations are concerned about estimates on the numbers of children potentially impacted by parental substance use and how to engage with them.

Awareness of trauma informed approaches is increasing and questions arise on the impact of domestic abuse or adverse childhood experiences on people who use drugs and their families. Globally there is a growing concern on how to inform the debate on cannabis policies and how to assess if the chosen policy will be acceptable to the general population.

The aim of this book is to provide researchers, service providers, and policy makers with a step-by-step guide with robust methodologies and illustrative case studies to address these challenges. The objective of each chapter is to answer a key question, provide a summary of the background evidence, demonstrate through a series of logical steps how to obtain local evidence, and finally illustrate the process with detailed, real-life case studies.

As addiction is encountered across a wide range of professions and civil society organizations, this book will be essential for graduate students of medicine, public health, addiction, psychology, and health and social care professions. It will be a guiding reference book for commissioners and providers of related policies and services. At a local level the step-by-step case studies will provide an easy-to-follow framework for those wishing to apply the methods to benefit and improve their own practice, service, or policy.

Contents

List of Figures

List of Tables

About the Author

Catherine Comiskey is a Professor in Healthcare Modelling and Statistics at the School of Nursing and Midwifery, Trinity College, Dublin University, Ireland. The School was ranked number 26 in the world by the QS subject ranking of 2024. Catherine holds a Ph.D. in biostatistics, biomathematics, and epidemiology. Within the School, Catherine has held positions of Head of School, Director of Research and Inaugural and Founding Director of the Trinity Centre for Practice and Healthcare Innovation. From 2020 to 2023 she was appointed as the inaugural Academic Director of the CHARM-EU Project (Challenge driven Accessible, Research led, Mobile, European University) and was the Chair of the International Academic Board and Academic Director of the Master's Program on Global Challenges for Sustainability.

Her research is in epidemiology and addiction. She was elected by her European peers as the Chair of the European Union's Scientific Committee of the EMCDDA, Lisbon (European Monitoring Centre for Drugs and Drug Addiction) 2020–2024, Vice-Chair from 2017 to 2020, and a member from 2014 to 2017. She is the ministerial appointed academic expert to the Irish National Drug Strategy Implementation Committee. She has acted as a consultant to the International Narcotics Control Board (INCB). She is the sole author of the book *Addiction Debates* published by Sage UK in 2020 and author of over 150 research papers in addiction, including work on estimates of prevalence, treatment outcomes, innovation; ageing and children of parents who use substances.

On a personal note, Catherine is married to Peter Carroll, an architect, they have four adult children, two elderly dogs, and a cat. She enjoys reading, walking, chatting with friends, and sea swimming.

Abbreviations

ACE	Adverse Childhood Experience
ACE	Adverse Community Environment
AI	Artificial Intelligence
AIDS	Acquired Immune Deficiency Syndrome
ANOVA	Analysis of Variance
AR	Augmented Reality
ASAM	American Society for Addiction Medicine
ASD	Autism Spectrum Disorder
ADHD	Attention Deficit Hyperactivity Disorder
BI	Brief Intervention
BMI	Body Mass Index
CAAN	Canadian Aboriginal Aids Network
CBT	Cognitive Behavioral Therapy
CDC	Centre for Disease Control and Prevention
CDI	Children's Depression Inventory
CDI	Childhood Development Initiative
CES	Centre for Effective Services
CFIR	Consolidated Framework for Implementation Research
C.I.	Confidence Interval
DARE	Drug Abuse Resistance Education
DAVINA	Domestic Abuse and Violence Is Never Acceptable
DAWN	Deaths Avoided With Naloxone
DNA	Did Not Attend
DORIS	Drug Outcome Research in Scotland
DL	Distributed Leadership
ECBI	Eyberg Child Behavior Inventory
EMCDDA	European Monitoring Centre for Drugs and Drug Addiction
ESPAD	European School Survey Project on Alcohol and Other Drugs
EUDA	European Drugs Agency
FRAMES	Feedback, Responsibility, Advice, Menu Options, Empathy and Self-Efficacy

GBL	Gamma Butyrolactone
GHB	Gamma Hydroxybutyrate
GHN	Gay Health Network
GHQ-28	General Health Questionnaire
GIF	Generic Implementation Framework
GMHS	Gay Men's Health Service
HAT	Healthy Addiction Treatment Recovery Model
HBV	Hepatitis B Virus
HCV	Hepatitis C Virus
HDG	Horizontal Drugs Group
HEARTS	Healthy Environments and Response to Trauma in Schools
HIV	Human Immunodeficiency Virus
HRBQ	Health Related Behaviour Questionnaire
HRQoL	Health Related Quality of Life
HTL	The Heart of Teaching and Learning
IBBS	Integrated Bio-behavioral Survey
ICD-10	International Classification of Diseases, Tenth Revision
IDU	intravenous drug use
IEG	Independent Evaluation Group
INCB	International Narcotics Control Board
INPUD	International Network of People Who Use Drugs
IOAD	International Overdose Awareness Day
IoT	Internet of Things
M&E	Monitoring and Evaluation
MARPS	Most at Risk Populations
MI	Motivational Interviewing
MOOC	Massive Open Online Course
MSM	Men who have Sex with Men
NHTC	New Haven Trauma Coalition
NIDA	National Institute of Drug Abuse
NIH	National Institute of Health
NPS	Novel Psychoactive Substances
OECD	Organization for Economic Co-operation and Development
OPS	Overdose Prevention Sites
ORC	Organizational Readiness for Change
OTI	Opiate Treatment Index
PDSA	Plan do Study Act
PEP	Post-exposure prophylaxis
PrEP	Pre-Exposure Prophylaxis
PRISM	Practical Robust Implementation Sustainability Model
PTSD	Post-Traumatic Stress Disorder
RAR	Rapid Assessment and Response
RCT	Randomized Control Trial
RDS	Respondent Driven Sampling
RE-AIM	Reach, Effectiveness, Adoption. Implementation and Maintenance

ROSIE	Research Outcome Study in Ireland Evaluating Drug Treatment Effectiveness
SAMHSA	Substance Abuse Mental Health Service Administration
SAOR	Support, Ask and Assess, Offer Assistance and Refer
SBCM	Strength-Based Case Management
SBEF	Strengths-Based Engagement Framework
SDG	Sustainable Development Goal
SDQ	Strengths and Difficulties Questionnaire
SIF	Safe Injection Facility
S-O-S	Stop Overdose Safely
STEEP	Social, Technological, Economic, Environmental and Political
SUD	Substance Use Disorder
STBBI	Sexually Transmitted Blood Borne Infection
STI	Sexually Transmitted Infection
TB	Tuberculosis
THN	Take Home Naloxone
TIP	Trauma Informed Practice
TIP	Treatment Improvement Protocol
TMFs	Theories, Models, and Frameworks
UNDRR	United Nations Office for Disaster Risk Reduction
UNGASS	United Nations General Assembly Special Session
UNODC	United Nations Office on Drugs and Crime
VR	Virtual Reality
VT	Vicarious Trauma
WCG	Washington Circle Group
WDR	World Drug Report
WRAP	Wellness Recovery Action Plan

Chapter 1
Introduction: What Challenges Are Policy and Practice Facing?

Challenging Times and Times of Opportunity

Now more than ever as policy makers and practitioners face both expected and unforeseen demands, the need for evidence-informed responses is crucial. As the global political and economic domains face increasing pressures, industries and services are at the forefront, leading and managing demands. Universal health insurance while a laudable goal, can only be sustained if policy and practice perform to meet the needs and improve health and well-being at the individual level. There exists a constant tension between addressing the urgent and the important, while also balancing the challenges which were expected with those that were not anticipated.

The aim of this book is to provide a succinct, yet comprehensive approach to obtaining the local evidence needed for a series of globally relevant challenges. Many of these challenges are ongoing and must be addressed on a regular basis as populations change and needs vary. The simplest of such questions one might ask is, "how many people need our service and what is the current prevalence?" While the prevalence of what or who may vary across a region or a time, the questions remain to be answered.

For example, we may ask, "how many people need our services while attending music festivals?" Equally we may ask, "how many children who are living with a parent who uses substances need support?" Other questions and challenges may emerge unexpectedly or because of a so-called disruptive innovation. These occurrences may bring new opportunities alongside the challenge. Examples of such could be, "given climate change concerns, how can we make our service more sustainable?" Or "how can our service take advantage of new technologies such as artificial intelligence, virtual realities or Chat GPT?" Or we might ask, "how can our service engage extra resources and respond to this unexpected disaster?" Many of these questions faced by policy and practice are addressed within this book.

C. Comiskey, *Addiction Research and Evaluation*, Advances in Mental Health and Addiction, https://doi.org/10.1007/978-3-031-65917-1_1

An Overview of Hot Topics and Challenges in Addiction

Challenges addressed include the ongoing challenge of developing evidence-informed policies. Within Chap. 2, we explore approaches to estimating the size of unknown populations. Globally it is estimated by the United Nations Office for Drugs and Crime (UNODC) World Drug Report 2023 (UNODC, 2023) that almost 300 million people used drugs in 2021. Yet we cannot tell how many older people there may be who are misusing their prescribed medications, or within some regions of the world how many people who use drugs are also HIV positive. Established and recommended methods for providing estimates for these types of hidden populations are provided within Chap. 2. Once we know the scale of our challenge, we move on in Chap. 3 to explore how we identify specific needs related to our client group.

In Chap. 4, we take a step back and address prevention and intervention and how to ensure we choose an effective and relevant program. Within the recent past there has been a vast increase in the number of prevention programs available for varying contexts. Yet often such programs remain untested and can lack adequate rigor in their design. Indeed, it has been found that poorly designed prevention programs can produce unintended consequences and can increase the use of substances.

In Chap. 5, we move forward to the next stage to examine the challenge of evaluation and ensuring our treatment or recovery program is fit for purpose and is having an impact both in terms of outcomes and processes. All too often treatment regimens have simply been handed down from practitioner to practitioner under the assertion, "this is how we have always done things here."

Within Chap. 6, we explore rapid assessment and responses to unplanned and emerging threats. This includes responding to disasters and community recovery. Within the recent past we have seen the need to respond urgently to unanticipated pandemics, unimaginable death tolls due to synthetic opioids and the movement of people across almost all continents because of war, military coups, earthquakes, and religious ideologies. Chapter 7 will continue the exploration of these topics with an emphasis on addressing increased mortality among some groups of peoples.

Chapter 8 addresses the enduring nature of stigma, across not only communities but also generations of families from infant to grandparent, many of whom have suffered needless additional harms and traumas as a result. We continue to witness stigma despite numerous United Nations conventions on human rights, the rights of children and the rights of those with disabilities. The opportunity a trauma-informed approach presents is also discussed in Chap. 8. Within this discussion we explore the need for distributed leadership and the principles of inclusivity, diversity, dignity, and respect within person-centered care.

Chapter 9 builds upon the evidence and approaches within the previous chapters with a focus on using the evidence to enable good policy. It describes how policy might be developed given the evidence, the recognition of the prevailing philosophies and the importance of distributed leadership and the co-design process.

Chapter 10 follows on from policy development and looks at implementation. It provides details on the opportunities that the tools and procedures of implementation science and monitoring and evaluation can bring to policy and service. The concept and requirements of readiness for change and scaling up are provided.

Chapter 11 concludes the book by looking forward to explores opportunities arising from disruptive innovations from basic telemedicine in resource poor settings to online consultations and from artificial intelligence to Chat GPT4 as tools for teaching and learning. Within this chapter we also explore how to engage these technologies to share learning on best practice across services. Finally, Chap. 11 also addresses the all too important question of climate change and asks how we can work towards and ultimately develop an environmentally ethical and sustainable addiction service that address the sustainable development goals and the ultimate challenge of One Health for people who use substances.

The One Health High-Level Expert Panel (OHHLEP), whose members represent a broad range of disciplines in science and policy-related sectors from around the world, updated the definition of One Health in 2021 (One Health Commission, 2023). The OHHLEP definition states that,

> One Health is an integrated, unifying approach that aims to sustainably balance and optimize the health of people, animals and ecosystems. It recognizes the health of humans, domestic and wild animals, plants, and the wider environment (including ecosystems) are closely linked and inter-dependent. The approach mobilizes multiple sectors, disciplines and communities at varying levels of society to work together to foster well-being and tackle threats to health and ecosystems, while addressing the collective need for clean water, energy and air, safe and nutritious food, taking action on climate change, and contributing to sustainable development.

This definition was endorsed internationally by the Food and Agriculture Organization of the United Nations (FAO), the World Organization for Animal Health (OIE), the United Nations Environment Programme (UNEP), and the World Health Organization (WHO) who established the advisory panel OHHLEP. Together, these organizations form the One Health Commission (One Health Commission, 2023) (see https://www.onehealthcommission.org/en/why_one_health/what_is_one_health/). One Health reinforces the ambitions of the SDGs and recognizes that good health depends on and contributes to other development goals, underpinned by a systems approach incorporating social justice, economic prosperity, and environmental protection (Dye, 2018, 2022). Within addiction research and evaluation, we will explore how this approach can aid the development of sustainable and effective policy, practices, and services.

Related Global Epidemiology and the Need for Evidence-Based Policy and Practice

The need to address the varying challenges can be seen when we explore the global epidemiology of substance use and the impact illegal drug production has on individuals, their communities, and the environment. According to the World Drug Report (2023) of the United Nations Office on Drugs and Crime (UNODC) (UNODC, 2023), in terms of the number of people who used drugs within 2021, this was estimated at over 296 million and this number had increased substantially over the past decade. The number of people who not only use drugs but also are diagnosed with suffering from a drug use disorder has increased by approximately 45% within the last decade and currently this is estimated at almost 40 million people.

Comparing this number of people with a drug use disorder with similar cancer data allows us to put the scale of these vast numbers in context. According to the World Cancer Research Fund International (2023), excluding skin cancers, there was an estimated 18 million people with cancer in 2020. Comparing these two numbers we can see that globally, there are more than double the numbers of people suffering from drug use disorders compared to the numbers diagnosed with cancer, yet only one in five people suffering from drug-related disorders were in treatment for drug use in 2021. A widening of the disparities in access to treatment across regions of the globe was also reported by the UNODC (UNODC, 2023).

A broad comparison of the scale of the treatment provision markets for both diagnoses highlight further the challenges facing policies and services for people who use drugs. According to Research and Markets (2023), the substance abuse treatment market size was estimated to be growing and was approximately $11.5 billion US dollars in 2022. The global oncology market was estimated by Precedence Research (2023) to be $203.5 billion US dollars in 2022. This cancer market size is over 17 times the substance abuse market size.

Research and Markets (2023) also notes that the treatment for substance use market is provided by hospitals, rehabilitation centers, clinics, and others but the hospital market is by far the largest accounting for over one third of the market. This dominant share of the hospital sector may be explained by the delay in seeking an early diagnosis and treatment due to societal stigma. The delay can also contribute to the development of additional medical conditions linked to the substance use such as cardiovascular disease, stroke, cancer, additional infectious diseases such as Hepatitis and finally mental disorders.

Behind each of these market statistics is a person who, because of this delay, is suffering more than they need to, a family who is worrying about their loved one, and a community who is at the loss of a contributing and participating individual. This challenge of stigma will be discussed in more detail in Chap. 8.

The scale of illicit drug markets of the European Union is explored jointly by Europol and the European Union Drug Agency (EUDA). In their EU drug markets report they highlight that illicit drugs account for around one fifth of global crime proceeds (EMCDDA and Europol, 2023). Within Europe cocaine is the second largest market after cannabis and its use is on the rise. It is estimated that the EU cocaine retail market was worth at least EUR 10.5 billion in 2020. Coca and cocaine production is reported to have become more efficient, and it continues to increase in South America and appears to have become more internationalized and includes efficient production in Europe. According to UNODC (2023) the drug economy in the Amazon Basin is exacerbating additional criminal activities and damaging the environment of the world's largest rainforest. According to the EMCDDA and Europol (2023) information exists to suggest that some Latin American and European criminal networks are partnering in cocaine production activities in Europe, and perhaps also in South America. This phenomenon has also been observed for other drugs, particularly methamphetamine. In terms of methamphetamine the drug ban in Afghanistan has decreased the opium poppy production with a loss of earning by local farmers. As Afghanistan is a major producer of methamphetamine the drop in opiate cultivation could drive a shift towards synthetic drug manufacture, where different actors will benefit at the loss of the local farmers.

Clearly the global epidemiology of substance use and the related markets is a complex system of winners and losers from faming families to large multinational medical or insurance corporations to global criminal networks. From individual people who may be sons or daughters, mothers or fathers who need treatment to teachers providing prevention messages or nations dealing with fentanyl crises. Within the next section we move forward and explore how we might simplify this complexity and identify and define our key challenge with a partnership approach.

Clarifying the Problem and Its Scope: Defining Your Research and Evaluation Questions

Defining your challenge and hence your research and evaluation question is a process. Research questions may be derived from clinical practice, from community observations or from personal experience. These different settings may point towards an unmet demand for certain needs assessments, for program evaluations or clinical effectiveness studies. Often however the research and evaluation question arise from personal practice and observation. For example, it may be the case that clients are not engaging with a service as it is not meeting their needs, or a program has been running within a service and has never been fully evaluated.

Perhaps a new need has emerged because of a national or international event or because of a change in public opinion. For example, there is currently a global paradigm shift in cannabis policies and ministries are re-evaluating their existing policies. Resources may have changed, perhaps cutbacks are required or perhaps there has been an unexpected increase in funding and decisions are needed on where best to allocate the extra monies.

Regardless of the origin of the challenge, an agreed key question with a related aim and objectives is required. The development of this question usually follows a pattern. The six stages in the development of a key question to address a challenge are outlined in Fig. 1.1.

Once the question has been finalized, it can be stated as an overarching aim of the study. To realize this aim, a series of related objectives each representing a further question and contributing to the overarching question and aim can be devised. The answer to each of these further questions collectively provide the answer to the overarching aim and hence the challenge. For example, a service might have a primary aim of evaluating their treatment regime. The related key question the service asks is: "Does our treatment work?" To help answer this question the service can pose several related questions based on their treatment goals. These may be, "Does treatment reduce the risk of overdose?"; "Does treatment reduce drug use?"; "Does treatment improve physical and mental health?". Once the general topic of enquiry is decided upon the next step is to work with the relevant stakeholders to develop and refine the aim and objectives and the related questions.

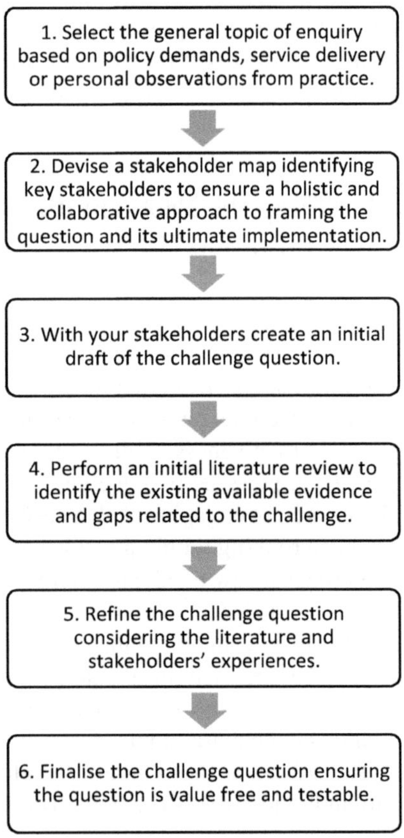

Fig. 1.1 The six stages in the development of a key question to address a challenge

Stakeholder Mapping and Engagement

The National Implementation Research Network (2023) provides an excellent resource to aid the identification of stakeholders and the role they play in addressing your challenge, your key research question or aim, and the related objectives.

The role stakeholders play can vary and range from:

- Co-creators who are critical to the project and share the leadership, decision-making, and actions to complete the work.
- Collaborators, who share in decision-making; those who you need to involve but do not contribute to decision-making.
- Those whom you can consult for feedback.
- Those partners whom you inform and who in turn inform others.

Figure 1.2 illustrates this.

The Centre for Effective Services (CES, 2017) provide a tool for stakeholder mapping and contribution based on what is referred to as a power matrix. An online example from Improvement Service Scotland (2023) is provided in Fig. 1.3. The power matrix is used for categorizing stakeholders during a change project to allow them to be effectively managed. Stakeholders are plotted on the grid in relation to the power and interest they have in respect of the project. The grid categorizes stakeholders into the following four groups:

- High power/high interest.
- High power/low interest.
- Low power/high interest.
- Low power/low interest.

Stakeholders with high power and interest need to be engaged with regularly and their input to the framing of the challenge is essential. However, stakeholders with low power but high interest are also crucial to ensure their needs and voices are

Importance of the challenge/question to the stakeholder	High	**Inform or consult**	**Collaborate or involve**
	Low	**Inform**	**Consult or involve**
		Low	High
		Influence of the stakeholder over the challenge/question	

Fig. 1.2 The level of engagement of stakeholders given their influence and the importance of the challenge question to them

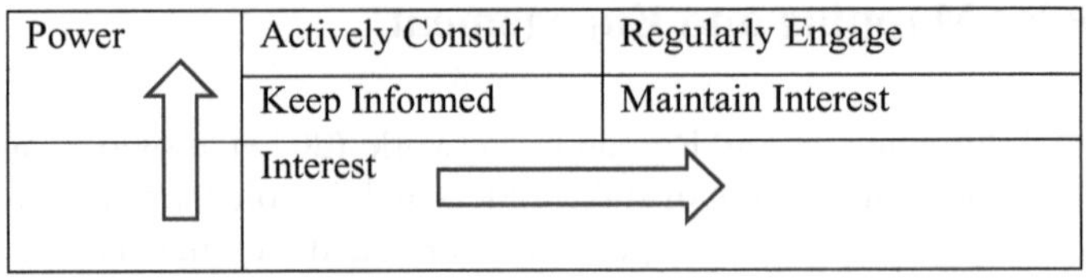

Fig. 1.3 Power interest grid

heard. Such stakeholders might represent people with experience of addiction or their family members.

Reviewing the Literature

Once a draft question representing the challenge is formulated it is important to review the national and international literature including what is known as grey literature, to identify if the question has been addressed by others and if so, what can be learned and what gaps in knowledge remain. The importance of, and the growth in the methodologies and types of literature reviews available has increased substantially in the recent past. Grant and Booth (2009) provided one of the first summaries of review types and this has been updated and extended by (Sutton et al., 2019). Brennan et al. (2020) have provided a succinct summary of key, but not all, review types. PhD on Track (2022) also provide a good outline on choosing a review type that will depend on the resources and time available and the nature of the review question. Combining these two resources to create an overall list of review types and is reproduced in Fig. 1.4.

The more specific the topic or question being searched is, the more focused the result will be. Cronin et al. (2008) provide a list of useful steps to follow in a review and steps common to most review types are provided below within the context of our stakeholder grouping.

1. Formulate the research question with the identified stakeholders.
2. Set realistic inclusion and exclusion criteria to ensure the review is achievable within the resources available.
3. Select and access the literature, this is a task that may need to be shared out among team members as the workload at this stage can be substantial. Relevant software such as Covidence systematic review software, Veritas Health Innovation, Melbourne, Australia, available at www.covidence.org. can be helpful.
4. Assess the quality of the literature included in the review. This step is not usually required within a rapid review. If it is required, then at least two reviewers are needed. One to appraise the quality and one to perform a check on the quality scores from either all or a selected sample of the included papers.

Type of review	Speed	Methodological detail	Risk of bias	Comprehensiveness
	Quick	Less	Increased	Less
Narrative				
Rapid				
Scoping				
Review of reviews				
Systematic quantitative				
Systematic qualitative				
Systematic integrative				
	Slow	More	Decreased	More

Fig. 1.4 Types of reviews adapted from Brennan et al. (2020) and PhD on Track (2022). (Online reference: https://www.ncbi.nlm.nih.gov/pmc/articles/PMC7333781/figure/F1/)

5. Analyze and synthesize the findings. This is usually done by the main reviewer but again, findings can be assessed by a second reviewer. The approach to the analysis and synthesis can vary depending on the level of expertise available within the team, the needs of the review and whether a meta-analysis is required. Braun and Clarke (2006) provide a very good overview from a simple content analysis looking at the frequency of topics across the included papers, to a top down, deductive analysis possibly using predefined criteria or a bottom up, inductive approach within the use of any pre-defined criteria.
6. Conclude on what is known about the challenge topic and key question and clarify where the gaps in the literature remain. This is an essential final step and is the overarching aim of the review.

Refining the Challenge Question

Once what is known and what the gaps in the literature are, the research question addressing the challenge can be finalized with the appropriate level of input from the stakeholders. At this stage the budget and resources may also need to be considered to ensure the chosen question is feasible in terms of resources. Guerin and Comiskey (2017) explore this and note that varying stakeholders may not have contributed equally both professionally and financially to the project, yet the researcher must be able to form the challenge question from the perspective of all stakeholders. They must also endeavor to identify from the literature review and stakeholder meetings the key question of greatest value and benefit to all involved taking the power matrix into consideration.

Jacobsen (2021) speaks of generating what she calls, *testable questions*. Testability according to Jacobsen is the ability of a research or challenge question to be answered using experiments or other types of measurements. A good research question is one that can end in a question mark and is not stating any value judgments. A research question should be value free, and the research developed may ultimately contribute towards understanding the value. For example, Jacobsen says you cannot have a statement such as, "Cannabis use is bad," even if this is framed as the question, "Is cannabis use bad?" This question cannot be answered as there is no scale to measure the concept of badness.

While value statements may arise during the early stages of devising the research challenge, such statements cannot be used as testable research questions and the subsequent informing of evidence-based practice. A value neutral, measurable, and more appropriate question may be, "Does parental cannabis use increase the risk of early onset cannabis use among the children of these parents?" Guerin and Comiskey (2017) explore the key research question in more depth.

Ethics and Good Research Practice Considerations

Ethical principles are grounded in a range of international declarations originating from the Nuremberg Code of 1947 which followed the Nuremberg trials (Leaning, 1996). This code established ten basic principles which were to be observed and which addressed moral, ethical, and legal concepts. It set out the need for voluntary-informed consent. The Declaration of Helsinki followed in 1964 and this declaration was adopted by the World Medical Association (World Medical Association, 1964). The declaration provided ethical principles for medical research involving human subjects (World Medical Association, 2023). Risks, burdens, and benefits to human subjects were specifically addressed as were vulnerable groups and individuals. The declaration also addressed scientific requirements and research protocols, the need for research ethics committees and it also addressed privacy and confidentiality concerns. The declaration also stipulated the need for the publication and dissemination of results and finally it noted that unproven interventions in clinical practice could be used for treatment where proven interventions did not exist.

The Belmont Report of 1979 (Department of Health and Human Services, 1979) extended previous international agreements and aimed to provide the basic ethical principles for the conduct of both biomedical and behavioral research (The National Commission for the Protection of Human Subjects of Biomedical and Behavioral Research, 1979). The report established three basic principles for the ethical conduct of human research these being, respect for persons, beneficence, and justice. These three principles remain the corner stone of all ethics committees today. However, while all are aware of the need for ethical clearance prior to starting a study, not many consider the concept of, Good Research Practice.

Throughout the process of addressing challenges within addiction services and policy, the need for good research practice is essential. Most practitioners and policy makers are aware of the need for strict ethical approvals and controls, but few may be aware of the general principles of good research practice. The appropriate governance of a project is essential, especially when working both with internal and external stakeholders with varying power balances as outlined in the stakeholder mapping exercise.

Good research practice is a culture and is not something that can be directly monitored. Good practice should permeate through the full research process spanning the research integrity and inclusivity processes, training, supervision, and mentoring of all staff involved, all aspects of the ethical approval process, the research data management and reporting of results processes and finally the publication practices. This list is not exhaustive and as new technologies and data gathering processing emerge such as data scraping of open-source websites or the use of artificial intelligence to assist with writing, the need for good governance and research practices will continue to be of the utmost importance to protect both the staff and the stakeholders and the integrity of the findings from the challenge addressed. The use of new technologies and disruptive innovation is discussed in more detail in Chap. 11.

A succinct summary with ten practical steps for good research practice within the research and reporting processes is provided by Schwab et al. (2022) in Switzerland. These include:

1. Specifying a research question, as detailed within this chapter.
2. Writing a study proposal or protocol. This is a summary document which outlines your full research plan.
3. Deciding on an appropriate sample size for your study. This will depend on the nature of your study and your study design. Details of this are covered within Chap. 5.
4. Developing a data management plan. This may be part of your ethical application or form part of your protocol or proposal. A data management plan outlines where the data will be stored, who will have access, how amendments to the database will be agreed and made if necessary.
5. Focus on reducing any potential bias within your research and stakeholders. For example, social desirability bias.
6. Be wary of unintentionally introducing bad research practices such as selective reporting of findings to support your theory or hypotheses.
7. Be prudent when reporting statistical significance especially when multiple tests are being conducted.
8. Where possible and ethical, provide open access to your data sources so that findings may be replicated by others.
9. Report all findings, both those that support and disagree with any of your hypotheses.

10. Report your finding in line with international reporting guidelines. A range of these can be found on the EQUATOR Network, see https://www.equator-network.org/ (Equator Network, 2023).

An example of good research practice with broad stakeholder engagement is provided in Case Study 1.1.

Case Study 1.1: Substance Use and Neurodiversity

Introduction

The World Health Organization describes neurodevelopmental disorders as behavioral and cognitive disorders that occur during a baby's developmental period: these include autism spectrum disorder and attention deficit hyperactivity disorder (ADHD) amongst others (WHO, 2023). ADHD according to the WHO is characterized by a persistent pattern of inattention and/or hyperactivity-impulsivity that has a direct negative impact on academic, occupational, or social functioning. Autism spectrum disorder (ASD) constitutes a diverse group of conditions characterized by some degree of difficulty with social communication and reciprocal social interaction, as well as persistent restricted, repetitive, and inflexible patterns of behavior, interests, or activities (WHO, 2023) (see https://www.who.int/news-room/fact-sheets/detail/mental-disorders).

This impairment-related description of ADHD and ASD is being challenged with the emerging concept of neurodiversity. Neurodiversity according to Neurodiversity Ireland (2023) describes the differences in the way people's brains work. There is no one or correct way for the brain to work and instead, there is a wide range of ways that people perceive and respond to the world. According to Neurodiversity Ireland the term was developed to overcome stigma and support people who are neurodivergent. This includes people with the most common neurotypes of ADHD, Autism, Dyslexia, Dyspraxia, Tourette's and Tics. As neurodivergent people experience, interpret and interact with the world in unique ways, the aim is to focus on an individual's strengths and talents and enable society to address challenges with inclusive creative problem-solving skills involving both neurodivergent and neurotypical people (Neurodiversity Ireland, 2023) (see https://neurodiversityireland.com/what-is-neurodiversity/).

Within the research literature on substance use, an increased prevalence of people with co-occurring neurodiversity and substance use disorder has been noted (Gujska et al., 2023). In spite of this emerging research, few international substance use polices address this challenge. A brief overview of the American, Canadian and Irish policy within a graduate course found that while mental health issues may sometimes be, but not always, noted within the policies, neurodiversity was omitted (private communication with Constanze Sophie Connearn, Stephen Downey, Ipo Kok, Helena Vitria Pujol and Britt Peters, CHARM-EU students at Trinity College

Dublin, June 2023). The Substance Abuse and Mental Health Service Administration of the U.S. Department of Health and Human Services has however provided an advisory on the topic (SAMHSA, 2015).

Methods

The INCAS study of the International Collaboration on ADHD and Substance Abuse (ICASA) foundation designed an International Naturalistic Cohort Study of ADHD and Substance Use Disorders Study (INCAS) to address this recognized gap (Brynte et al., 2022).

Results

Within their work we can see in Table 1.1 how, within their study, the initial steps for good research practice were followed. It remains to be seen if the full study when published will continue this practice.

Discussion

Since the publication of the INCAS study, an international consensus statement for the screening, diagnosis and treatment of adolescents with concurrent ADHD and SUD has been developed (Özgen et al., 2020). This consensus statement was a good example of stakeholder engagement as it involved experts from 55 agencies across 17 countries including young people agencies. Consensus was reached across the stakeholders on 36 of 37 statements across six domains on screening, diagnosis, and treatment.

To conclude, within this chapter we have seen that given the global and local epidemiology and drug markets, many challenges exist within addiction services and policies. However, not all can be addressed initially. There is a need to identify, potentially initially from practice what appears to be the most urgent challenge area that needs to be addressed. Mapping your stakeholders and their role and inviting them to contribute to the refinement of the broad challenge is the next step. Once the main challenge has been decided there is a need then to review the literature and assess if the literature has already addressed this or if a gap remains. The full team of stakeholders can then refine the challenge question is light of the evidence. How to address specific challenges is the topic of the subsequent chapters. Across all this process, we promote and develop and ensure a culture of good research practice and remember to enjoy the journey and the findings.

Table 1.1 Initial good research practice steps for the INCAS study of ADHD and substance use disorders. (Brynte et al., 2022)

Initial good research practice steps	
Good research practice	Evidence of this step being addressed within the study
Specifying a research question	"The aims of this … study is to describe the treatment modalities provided to individuals with SUD + ADHD entering SUD treatment, and to identify predictors of successful treatment outcomes, as measured by retention in treatment, the reduction in substance use and ADHD symptoms and the global functioning at 3 and 9-months follow-up"
Writing a study proposal or protocol. This is a summary document which outlines your full research plan	The trial protocol is written and registered and publicly available at https://doi.org/10.1186/ISRCTN15998989 Trial registration: ISRCTN15998989 20/12/2019.
Deciding on an appropriate sample size	"Given the non-interventional observational design, the targeted sample size of enrolling 600 participants is not based on statistical power, but rather on the goal of providing a solid description of the specific patient population and variation in treatment modalities and clinical course."
Developing a data management plan	"In the current paper baseline characteristics are presented. In future publications additional analyses of baseline predictors, as independent variables of the main outcomes (retention to treatment, substance use as measured by TLFB, and ASRS score) as dependent variables, will be performed through survival analysis, regression models and mixed effect models. Other inferential statistical analyses will be considered using both univariate and multivariate models and considering the naturalistic (non-randomized) nature of the study using propensity score methods."
Focus on reducing any potential bias within your research and stakeholders	"…the treatments are not blinded nor randomly allocated, thus causing inferential challenges and difficulties in controlling for selection and information bias and/or confounding."
Be wary of unintentionally introducing bad research practices such as selective reporting of findings to support your theory or hypotheses	Evidence not available within this paper
Be prudent when reporting statistical significance especially when multiple tests are being conducted	Within this paper initial descriptive statistics are provided to describe the baseline characteristics of the participants
Where possible and ethical, provide open access to your data sources so that findings may be replicated by others	The datasets used are available from the corresponding author on reasonable request and this is stated within the paper

(continued)

Table 1.1 (continued)

Report all findings, both those that support and disagree with any of your hypotheses	As this is the baseline data no hypotheses are tested
Report your finding in line with international reporting guidelines	It is not stated within the paper if the STROBE guidelines for reporting observational studies was followed

References

Braun, V., & Clarke, V. (2006). Using thematic analysis in psychology. *Qualitative Research in Psychology, 3*(2), 77–101. https://doi.org/10.1191/1478088706qp063oa

Brennan, M. L., Arlt, S. P., Belshaw, Z., Buckley, L., Corah, L., Doit, H., Fajt, V. R., Grindlay, D. J., Moberly, H. K., & Morrow, L. D. (2020). Critically appraised topics (CATs) in veterinary medicine: Applying evidence in clinical practice. *Frontiers in Veterinary Science, 7*, 314.

Brynte, C., Aeschlimann, M., Barta, C., Begeman, A. H. A., Bäcker, A., Crunelle, C. L., Daigre, C., De Fuentes-Merillas, L., Demetrovics, Z., Dom, G., López, L. G., Icick, R., Johnson, B., Joostens, P., Kapitány-Fövény, M., Karsinti, E., Kiefer, F., Konstenius, M., Levin, F. R., et al. (2022). The clinical course of comorbid substance use disorder and attention deficit/hyperactivity disorder: protocol and clinical characteristics of the INCAS study. *BMC Psychiatry, 22*(1), 625.

CES. (2017). *Stakeholder engagement tool*. Centre for Effective Services. Retrieved May 23, 2023 from https://effectiveservices.notion.site/Stakeholder-Engagement-Tool-ee9e42366f644197ae5856457dff96bb

Cronin, P., Ryan, F., & Coughlan, M. (2008). Undertaking a literature review: A step-by-step approach. *British Journal of Nursing, 17*(1), 38–43.

Department of Health and Human Services. (1979). *The Belmont report: Ethical principles and guidelines for the protection of human subjects of research*. National Commission for the Protection of Human Subjects of Biomedical.

Dye, C. (2018). Expanded health systems for sustainable development. *Science, 359*(6382), 1337–1339.

Dye, C. (2022). One health as a catalyst for sustainable development. *Nature Microbiology, 7*(4), 467–468.

EMCDDA and Europol. (2023). *EU drug markets: In-depth analysis*. Retrieved August 28, 2023 from https://www.emcdda.europa.eu/publications/eu-drug-markets_en

Equator Network. (2023). *Toolkits: Reporting guidelines for main study types*. Enhancing the QUALity and Transparency Of health Research. https://www.equator-network.org/toolkits/

Grant, M. J., & Booth, A. (2009). A typology of reviews: An analysis of 14 review types and associated methodologies. *Health Information & Libraries Journal, 26*(2), 91–108.

Guerin, S., & Comiskey, C. (2017). Developing a detailed design for research with communities. In *Research and evaluation in community, health and social care settings* (pp. 77–89). Routledge.

Gujska, J. H., Silczuk, A., Madejek, R., & Szulc, A. (2023). Exploring the link between attention-deficit hyperactivity disorder and cannabis use disorders: A review. *Medical Science Monitor: International Medical Journal of Experimental and Clinical Research, 29*, e939749–e939741.

Improvement Service Scotland. (2023). *Introduction to the power/interest grid*. Retrieved May 26, 2023 from https://www.improvementservice.org.uk/business-analysis-framework/consider-perspectives/powerinterest-grid

Jacobsen, K. H. (2021). *Introduction to health research methods* (3rd ed.). Jones and Bartlett Learning.

Leaning, J. (1996). *War crimes and medical science* (Vol. 313, pp. 1413–1415). British Medical Journal Publishing Group.

Neurodiversity Ireland. (2023). *What is neurodiversity*. Retrieved August 28, 2023 from https://neurodiversityireland.com/what-is-neurodiversity/

One Health Commission. (2023). *What is one health?* https://www.onehealthcommission.org/en/why_one_health/what_is_one_health/

Özgen, H., Spijkerman, R., Noack, M., Holtmann, M., Schellekens, A. S., Van De Glind, G., Banaschewski, T., Barta, C., Begeman, A., & Casas, M. (2020). International consensus statement for the screening, diagnosis, and treatment of adolescents with concurrent attention-deficit/hyperactivity disorder and substance use disorder. *European Addiction Research, 26*(4–5), 223–232.

Precedence Research. (2023). *Oncology Market (By Cancer Di-agnostics & Treatment: Cancer Diagnostics and Cancer Treatment; By Indication: Lungs Cancer, Colorectal Cancer, Breast Cancer, Liv-er Cancer, Bladder Cancer, Head & Neck Cancer, Prostate Cancer, and Others) – Global Industry Analysis, Size, Share, Growth, Trends, Regional Outlook, and Forecast 2023–2032*. Retrieved August 28, 2023 from https://www.precedenceresearch.com/oncology-mar-ket#:~:text=The%20global%20oncology%20market%20was,total%20market%20share%20in%202021.

Research and Markets. (2023). *Substance abuse treatment global market report 2023: Sector to grow by 8.65% annually through* 2033 *with rising public awareness and increasing drug misuse boosting sector*. Retrieved August 28, 2023 from https://www.globenewswire.com/en/news-release/2023/03/16/2628555/28124/en/Substance-Abuse-Treatment-Global-Market-Report-2023-Sector-to-Grow-by-8-65-Annually-Through-2033-With-Rising-Public-Awareness-and-Increasing-Drug-Misuse-Boosting-Sector.html

SAMHSA. (2015). *Adults with attention deficit hyperactivity dis-order and substance use disorders*. Substance Abuse and Mental Health Services Administration. Retrieved September 1, 2023 from https://store.samhsa.gov/sites/default/files/d7/priv/sma15-4925.pdf

Schwab, S., Janiaud, P., Dayan, M., Amrhein, V., Panczak, R., Palagi, P. M., Hemkens, L. G., Ramon, M., Rothen, N., & Senn, S. (2022). *Ten simple rules for good research practice* (Vol. 18, p. e1010139). Public Library of Science.

Sutton, A., Clowes, M., Preston, L., & Booth, A. (2019). Meeting the review family: Exploring review types and associated information retrieval requirements. *Health information & libraries journal, 36*(3), 202–222. https://doi.org/10.1111/hir.12276

The National Commission for the Protection of Human Subjects of Biomedical and Behavioral Research. (1979). *The Belmont report: Ethical principles and guidelines for the protection of human subjects of research*. Retrieved August 31, 2023, from https://www.hhs.gov/ohrp/sites/default/files/the-belmont-report-508c_FINAL.pdf

UNODC. (2023). *United Nations Office on drugs and crime: World drug report 2023*. United Nations. Retrieved August 2, 2023 from https://www.unodc.org/unodc/en/press/releases/2023/June/unodc-world-drug-report-2023-warns-of-converging-crises-as-illicit-drug-markets-continue-to-expand.html?testme

WHO. (2023). *Mental disorders*. World Health Organization. https://www.who.int/news-room/fact-sheets/detail/mental-disorders

World Medical Association. (1964). *World Medical Association (1964) WMA declaration of Helsinki – Ethical principles for medical research involving human subjects*. Retrieved August 31, 2023 from https://www.wma.net/policies-post/wma-declaration-of-helsinki-ethical-principles-for-medical-research-involving-human-subjects/

World Medical Association. (2023). *The declaration of Helsinki: Medical research involving human subjects (2013)*. Retrieved December 1, 2023 from https://www.wma.net/what-we-do/medical-ethics/declaration-of-helsinki/

Chapter 2
Prevalence: What Is the Nature and Scale of the Problem?

Setting the Scene

"Gosh," said Anabel as she walked out of her consulting room. "Did you notice that we seem to have an increase in the number of women seeking information on domestic abuse?" she remarked to John as she passed the reception desk.

"That's interesting you should say that" John replied. "I've just had a phone call from a lady with three children who has asked if we can provide any services or recommendations for women seeking refuge." "Maybe we should put this down as item number one for our next planning meeting" responded Annabel as she scanned the faces of those waiting to enter her office for their weekly appointment. "I certainly noticed that there has been an increase, we really need to take a closer look at that."

"I agree," said John, "particularly given the complication of.., you know.., women who are using substances. It's so difficult for them trying to manage both their substance use and their children within a potentially abusive environment." "Ok", agreed Annabel as she wearily returned to her office, "let's try and do something about this and see if the numbers we're observing here in the clinic can be measured and how many more women might need our support."

As Anabel turned to walk back into her office, she caught sight of a discrete nod of approval from Trisha, a long-time service user, whose own mother had endured an abusive relationship. Anabel's weariness lifted as she called the next client and thought, "yes, that was the right decision."

C. Comiskey, *Addiction Research and Evaluation*, Advances in Mental Health and Addiction, https://doi.org/10.1007/978-3-031-65917-1_2

Introduction: The Challenge of Counting

Knowing the scale of the problem so that a service can be developed is one of the first challenges in the planning process. Asking the question, "how many?" is one of the simplest questions to pose, but it can also be one of the hardest questions to answer with certainty. Fortunately, this challenge has been addressed previously in varying circumstances with a range of approaches (UNODC, 2003). Within this chapter, we provide a step-by-step guide to each of these. The approaches presented have differing levels of complexity. The choice of which method to use can be based on the level of expertise available either in-house or otherwise, and the differing datasets that may be accessible. In addition, a service interested in estimating prevalence can also start with a simple case finding approach and then seek to build upon this as more information becomes available. With all the solutions presented, the need for appropriate local or national ethical approval, data protection procedures, and good research practice are essential.

Defining Prevalence: Specifying What It Is You Wish to Count

In its simplest form, prevalence may be defined as the number of exiting cases at a defined point in time within a defined region.

For example, we may wish to know the number of people over the age of 18 years using opioids within a city boundary in the year 2023. Similarly, we may wish to know the number (prevalence) of grandparents who have a grandchild with a parent who uses drugs living with them during the school year period. Related to this we may wish to know the number of children in a defined local region living with at least one parent who has a diagnosis of substance use disorder in the previous calendar year. To address any of these challenges it is important to first estimate the scale or the prevalence of the numbers so that services can be planned to meet the quantified need.

Related to prevalence is what is known as the prevalence rate. Two regions may have similar prevalence numbers, but their rates may be quite different. For example, the city of Rome in Italy may have a prevalence estimate of approximately 14,000 people using heroin in 1996 and the city of Dublin in Ireland may also have an estimate of approximately 14,000 people using heroin in the same year. However, the prevalence rate within Rome may be much lower than that of Dublin as the population size of Rome is far greater than that of Dublin (EMCDDA, 2002).

The prevalence rate allows us to compare regions or challenges and potentially prioritize which challenge is the greater and may need resources more urgently. For example, within a single city the prevalence of people who are hospitalized because of an overdose may be higher among those who have stable accommodation as opposed to those who are homeless. This number may be higher because the homeless population size may be lower. The prevalence rate of hospitalization from an overdose may however be much higher among people who are homeless as opposed to those who have the stable accommodation. While both challenges are extremely urgent, if resources are very scarce a decision may be made to address overdosing within the homeless population first as their prevalence rate is higher. They have a greater risk of hospitalization and potential death because of an overdose.

The prevalence rate is obtained by dividing the prevalence number within the defined group with the defined characteristic of interest by the total population size of that group. In our overdose example above the prevalence rate of hospitalization from overdose within the stable home population who use drugs in the last calendar year is given by:

- The number of people with a stable home who use drugs who were hospitalized in the last calendar year because of an overdose / The total number of people with a stable home and who use drugs in the last calendar year.
- If we know we have 12,000 people registered as using drugs and have stable accommodation in a region in the last year and if we know that in the last year 60 of these 12,000 people were hospitalized from an overdose, then the prevalence rate is given by 60/12,000 = 0.005.
- To enable us to interpret this number more easily we can multiply it by 100 and this allow us to express it as a percentage. We have, $0.005 \times 100 = 0.5\%$ or half of one percent.

The prevalence rate of hospitalization from overdose within the homeless population who use drugs in the last calendar year is given by:

- The number of homeless people who use drugs who were hospitalized in the last calendar year because of an overdose / The total number of people who were homeless and who used drugs in the last calendar year.
- If we know we have 800 people registered as homeless in a region in the last year who use drugs and if we know that in the last year 20 of these 800 people were hospitalized because of an overdose, then the prevalence rate is given by 20/800 = 0.025.
- Multiplying this result by 100 gives us, $0.025 \times 100 = 2.5\%$ or two and a half percent.

In the example above, we can see that the prevalence of hospitalization due to an overdose within the stable accommodation population was 60 people and within the homeless population it was 20. There were three times as many hospitalizations within the population with stable homes. However, when we look at the prevalence rates within the two population, we can see that the hospitalization rate from an overdose was five times higher within the homeless population as opposed to those with stable accommodation.

As the rates were both calculated in the same way and follow the same definition, they allow us to compare the two populations. The calculations demonstrate that while the prevalence number is higher within those with homes, the prevalence rate is higher within the homeless population. They are at greater risk and because of this they may need to be prioritized initially as part of an overall campaign.

To conclude, the prevalence rate describes the proportion of people in a population who have a defined challenge over a defined period within a defined geographical region. Calculating the prevalence rate for the same challenge for different groups allows us to compare between groups and can assist with deciding which group should take priority.

Similarly, if we estimate the prevalence rates for different challenges within a group, we can use these rates to set priorities for targeted actions within the group. We can see from this and from the example discussed above how powerful and useful prevalence estimation can be.

The five components for a prevalence definition are presented in Fig. 2.1.

Prevalence estimation can be obtained by both direct and indirect methods. A selection of these methods is provided.

Direct Method 1: Case Finding and Multisource Enumeration

Once the specific challenge, population, time frame, and location are clearly defined the simplest approach to prevalence estimation is case finding across several different sources of information. The objective with this task is to identify duplicates and remove them to avoid double counting. Where unique and anonymized identifiers and data sharing protocols exist, this makes this task much easier. However, this is seldom the case.

Where unique identifiers are not common across data sources one can be developed. For example, if each treatment center within the defined region agrees to provide a listing of unique cases based on initials, date of birth and expressed gender. The team addressing the challenge can receive the listing from each individual treatment center and remove people appearing more than once (see Table 2.1). We shall see how this approach was used in our case study on estimating the number of children with a parent who uses drugs and is receiving treatment.

This code for collecting the data is shared with each individual treatment center providing a data source. But it is not shared with the central person who is doing the

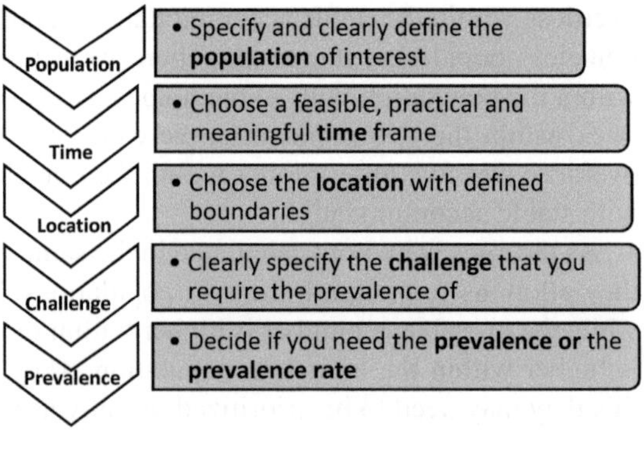

Fig. 2.1 Five components for a prevalence definition

Table 2.1 A unique code generator

First name initial	Surname initial	Day of birth	Month of birth	Year of birth	Gender initial

Table 2.2 Unique generated identifier codes A

Unique identifier codes from treatment center A. There are five cases within this center	
1	JB01051985M
2	CD12081992F
3	ZMcK31112001M
4	AM15012005M
5	SP17031993M

Table 2.3 Unique generated identifier codes B

Unique identifier codes from treatment center B. There are three cases within this center	
1	pZ05041999M
2	GB-L23122002M
3	KK15101998F

Table 2.4 Unique generated identifier codes C

Unique identifier codes from treatment center C. There are six cases within this center	
1	PC17041959M
2	GK23061960F
3	CC-C16111962F
4	AC13071970M
5	SP17031993M
6	LB24121973M

count and removing duplicates from the lists received across the sources. The central person receiving the lists of data is not aware of the code used to create the unique identifiers. In this code first initials of the names are suggested these could be changed to the second or the third initial. The format of the date of birth could also be changed to place the year of birth first for example.

The tables (Tables 2.2, 2.3, and 2.4) illustrate this approach. We can see from the tables that although there appears to be 5 + 3 + 6 = 14 cases across the three centers of the region. Centers A and C appear to have both counted the client with the unique identifier SP17031993M. Removing this client from the count gives a more accurate estimate of the true prevalence. We confirm that using a multisource estimation approach, the prevalence is 13 cases within the region of the three centers. This approach works well when numbers are small and centers are willing to prepare the data for the count.

The following tables (Tables 2.2, 2.3, and 2.4) list the generated identifiers for the people attending the three treatment centers within the time frame and region defined in the prevalence study.

Double Blinding the Code and the Count

With a multisource enumeration each data source provider prepares their own listing of cases from their records. The workload for compiling each individual list is spread across the owners of each of the data sources. The separate lists are not shared across sources but are shared with the central person in charge of the count. The person in charge of the count has no additional information. Indeed, they do not need to know how each part of the unique code is constructed. They merely check for duplicates across the data sources. The person in charge of devising the code does not need to see the lists generated from each source. By keeping the derived lists confidential from the code creator and by keeping the code construction confidential from the person counting and removing the duplicates, a double-blind approach can be achieved.

Multisource enumeration can be inexpensive and easily completed within a smaller region where agencies holding data sources may have good collaborative relationships. It may not be suitable for larger regions unless they already have a unique identifier and centralized database system in operation. Its key limitation in both larger and smaller regions is that it only counts cases already known to services. It does not capture hidden and unknown cases that may exist in the community and have unmet needs. A further limitation is that the code chosen for each person may not necessarily be unique. For example, more than one person may share the same initials, expressed gender and date of birth. General population surveys can help address this limitation. Similarly, there are more advanced methods that can be used to estimate prevalence of a hidden population as we shall see presently.

Direct Method 2: General Population Surveys

One of the traditional and most familiar methods used to estimate the prevalence of drug use in a population is a survey based on random sampling of the population concerned. This method has been widely used within localities and countries. When an inter-country comparison is required, this method proves costly to administer and difficult to ensure comparability of case definition. An example where this limitation has been successfully addressed is the European School Survey Project on Alcohol and Other Drugs (ESPAD, 2019). Using an agreed common protocol across 35 countries and 100,000 school children, an estimate of the prevalence of the use of cigarettes, alcohol, illicit drugs, inhalants, new psychoactive substances, and pharmaceuticals was obtained. The report also gathered information on gambling, the use of social media, and gaming.

As a common protocol was used across all countries, a comparison of prevalence rates could be obtained. For example, in terms of e-cigarette use it was found that on average, 14% of students in ESPAD countries had used e-cigarettes during the last 30 days. In 11 countries the last 30-day prevalence was less than 10%, with the lowest prevalence was observed in Serbia (5.4%). The highest rate was found in Monaco (41%), followed by Lithuania (31%) and Poland (30%) (ESPAD, 2019, p. 44). In general, when looking at the use of e-cigarettes within the last 30 days boys (16%) used more frequently than girls (11%). Iceland was the only country where the last 30-day prevalence of e-cigarette use was slightly higher among girls than boys (18% for girls versus 15% for boys) (ESPAD, 2019, p. 44).

General population surveys as the name suggests are useful for investigating the prevalence of an event or condition within a more general population. They are not useful for estimating the prevalence of rarer events or conditions. As the condition is rare and the sample generated is random, the sample may not find any or only a few cases of the rare condition. For example, if we wish to estimate the number of people who are in treatment for smoking heroin and have symptoms of active TB then a general population survey would not be appropriate. However, a survey of a random sample of people in treatment for smoking heroin among all the national treatment centers would be useful.

An example of a general population survey to estimate the prevalence of infectious diseases among a prison population was conducted by Allwright et al. (2000). Golrokhi et al. (2018) provide an extensive global review of the HIV prevalence and correlations in prisons in different regions of the world. When a general population survey is to be undertaken it is important that an adequate sample size is chosen and that the sample is chosen at random. To decide on what sample size may be needed a reputable online power calculator can be used with additional expert advice.

Indirect Method 1: Benchmark Multiplier Method

Multisource enumeration and general population surveys are known as direct methods of estimation as they involve using sources of data that directly capture the phenomena of interest be that drug use, TB treatment, HIV status, e-cigarette smoking or other substance use. It is often the case that a population is very hidden for several reasons, ranging from fear of stigma to fear of incarceration or similar. One such example is the fear of being diagnosed with what is known as a notifiable disease. For public health reasons it is obligatory to notify central record systems of many infectious disease. These include childhood diseases such as measles or rubella for example. They also include some infections that may, in the past, have been stigmatized such as HIV/AIDs, TB, Hepatitis C, and others.

Similarly, as was the case initially with the COVID-19 pandemic, many people may not know that they are infectious and may have no symptoms (Comiskey et al., 2021). Such cases are known as asymptomatic cases. When an infection can produce both asymptomatic and symptomatic cases the identification of the numbers infected becomes more challenging. The estimate of this hidden prevalence is required to enable the planning of a vaccination strategy, decisions on when a community has reached its critical threshold points and when policy makers and planners can advise on possible needle exchange service openings, overdose prevention sites and protection of multiple vulnerable communities.

When an infectious disease or a behavior such as substance use or injecting of a substance is hidden, then an alternative approach to prevalence estimation must be taken. Without the resources to find, test and enumerate asymptomatic infectious people or people with hidden behaviors then indirect estimation methods must be used. These have been used successfully internationally to produce estimates of the scale of a hidden infected population with HIV/AIDS or the scale of heroin use or the number of parents who use substances.

One such method is the benchmark multiplier method which is recommended by the European Drugs Agency (formerly known as the European Monitoring Centre for Drugs and Drug Addiction) for the estimation of the hidden numbers of people who use drugs (EMCDDA, 2004). In the context of problem drug use the total population of people who use drugs, given by T is unknown (partly hidden population). Given a sample of size B of the population in question (benchmark) and the probability c for someone of this unknown population to be member of the sample, the total population T can be estimated from.

$T = B$ divided by the probability of being in the population $1/c$ (this is the same as multiplying B by c) where B is the number of identified people who use drugs (sample or benchmark) and c is a parameter giving the probability of a drug user (unknown target population) to be a member of the identified sample B.

For example, if we know that we have 1500 people in treatment for injecting drug use, we say the benchmark $B = 1500$. If we also know from other studies or the international literature that between 20% and 25% (that is one fifth (1/5) to one quarter (1/4)) of people who inject drugs are in treatment, then this is our multiplier. We can then estimate that the true number of people who inject drugs is somewhere between.

$T = 1500$ multiplied by $5 = 7500$ and.
$T = 1500$ multiplied by $4 = 6000$.

We can then estimate that the true prevalence of people who inject drugs within the region and the time frame we have gathered the data, is between 6000 and 7500 people. This method does have its limitations due to its simplicity. The key limitation is the assumption of the linear relationship between prevalence of injecting and probability of being in treatment.

Substance use is also a complex challenge and many other local and regional factors, for example, mode of administration of the substance used, gender, age, access to treatment may also influence the linearity assumption. In addition, government policy and procedures on treatment notifications may delay or distort the number in the benchmark. As a result of these limitations, it is possible for the method to underestimate the true prevalence. The wide applicability of this method is illustrated in Case Study 2.1.

Indirect Method 2: Multivariate Indicator Method

To use the multiple indicator method to estimate prevalence for a region, data on each of the indicators used must be available for areas within the region. In addition, for at least two areas within the region there must be existing prevalence estimates. For example, if we wish to estimate the prevalence for a country, we must have estimates of prevalence for at least two regions in the country and data on indicators of substance use must be available in other regions in the country. The data collection period should also be the same for all the regions.

The following variables may be selected as indicators:

A. The number of offenses against drug laws or people who use drugs and who are in jail.
B. The number of drug-related deaths.
C. The number of clients in treatment.
D. The number of cases of AIDS related to intravenous drug use.
E. The number of hospital discharges for substance use.

In addition, the population size *F* of the population at risk is needed. This population at risk could be defined as a certain age group, for example adults over 18 and under 65 years old living in the country, in the year selected for the study. As stated, for at least two regions reliable estimates, *G* (maybe resulting from a previous study) are also necessary. These regions are called anchor points.

A simple yet comprehensive description of this method is provided by Comiskey (2001) and by Mollica and Mariani in EMCDDA (2001). To apply the method some statistical expertise is required. The method assumes a linear relationship between the unobserved prevalence and the observed indicators.

Indirect Method 3: The Capture Recapture Method

Hay and Richardson (2016) provide a review of the capture recapture method for estimating the hidden prevalence of substance use. They explain that the need for tackling intravenous substance use and the rise in HIV and AIDs cases in the 1980s and 1990s provided an impetus for the development of the method beyond its previous use in fisheries and ecological applications. As with these former applications, the method relies on capturing or marking people within one sample and then seeking to find how many of these marked or captured people can be found in a second sample. This can be repeated with two, three or more samples. The samples used with substance use epidemiology may be lists of people in treatment, list of people with a criminal record for drug possession or lists of people discharged from hospital for their substance use. As with other methods discussed, the lists must refer to the same geographic region, time frame, and defined population.

The method has been used most often to estimate the prevalence, that is, number of people using substances within a city in a defined year. By counting the number of people "captured" in three, two, and one sample the number not captured within any of the samples can be estimated using statistical modelling. Varying models can be fitted, from one that assumes that all the datasets are independent to one that includes dependencies between one or more datasets. Once the hidden population size is estimated it can be added to the known population once the duplicates have been removed and an estimate of the total population size can be derived. The choice of which model to apply and use for the estimation can depend on the nature of the datasets, the known epidemiology in the region and on the best model fit. In practice a range of models are fitted, and various estimates are produced. Figure 2.2 illustrates how three datasets might overlap.

As with all prevalence estimation methods there are a range of assumptions that must be met for the method to be applied. It is assumed that the population of people using drugs does not change during the period the prevalence is estimated. People do not begin or stop using drugs in the period and do not move in or out of the geographic region during the period the prevalence is estimated. It is assumed that people who use drugs can be identified within each source. That is, the overlaps can be measured. For example, if being in hospital for a long period of time may preclude one from obtaining a criminal record. Or if one is automatically sent for treatment when one is found in possession of drugs then the criminal record lists could be simply a subset of the treatment list. A full description of the assumptions and details of the application of the statistical methods are provided by Hay and Richardson (2016) and are outside the scope of this text.

Two case studies illustrating some of the methods discussed within this chapter are provided.

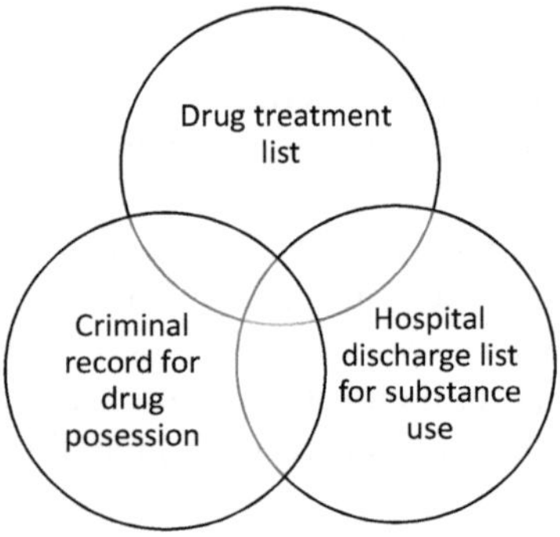

Fig. 2.2 Illustrating the potential overlaps in a three sample capture recapture study used to estimate the prevalence of substance use

Case Study 2.1: Estimating the Size of a Population Most at Risk of HIV/AIDS Using the Benchmark Multiplier Method

Introduction

Globally assessing the scale or the size of populations most at risk of acquiring HIV/AIDS and other infectious diseases is essential for the planning and provision of services. Within one country in the Balkans in central southeastern Europe, the Republic of Serbia devised a plan for monitoring and evaluation of the strategic response to HIV infection and AIDS for the country between 2011 and 2015. The plan set targets for HIV/AIDS prevention and one of the first priorities was to provide estimates of the scale of defined risk groups to be reached and targeted for intervention and prevention across various regions of the country. These Most at Risk Populations (MARPS) included people who injected drugs, people who worked in the sex industry, and men who had sex with men. The case study for people who inject drugs within the capital city of Belgrade is provided here. Belgrade has a population of almost 1.4 million people and is one of the oldest, continuously inhabited cities in Europe and the world.

Methods

To estimate the size of the population of people who inject drugs the benchmark multiplier method was used. To obtain estimates of an appropriate multiplier, a cross-sectional standardized integrated bio-behavioral survey (IBBS) was conducted within the city. The IBBS is an integrated biological and behavioral survey, seroprevalence data and data on the background information of the study participants, their knowledge, and their risk behaviors were collected. Respondents were contacted in the field or at treatment centers and interviewed by researchers trained to work on the project. RDS (respondent-driven sampling) and a snowball sampling strategy were used starting in locations where respondents were known by service providers to frequent. The snowball sample and the data from the survey was then used to form the multipliers.

The inclusion criteria for intravenous drug use (IDU) were for people aged 18 and more who injected a drug at least once in the last month and lived in the city for at least the last 3 months. The time periods for inclusion were chosen to reflect the different definitions of the risk. For example, within a drug using population, a person who may have injected almost a year ago may not be considered an active intravenous drug user, hence the inclusion criteria were injected within the last month. To ensure the final estimate produced was credible it was important to be aware of these minor yet important details.

Similarly, to ensure enough respondents were included to enable an estimate to be produced, a power analysis was conducted which found that 380 participants were required. The study received formal ethical approval from the Institute of Public Health of Serbia. All clients participating in the Integrated Bio-behavioral Surveillance Survey (IBBS) provided signed informed consent. The usual Wald confidence interval for a proportion was used to provide confidence intervals for the estimates of the multipliers.

Results

A total of 571 people who had injected within the last month responded to the survey in the two cities of Belgrade and Nis. In the two cities over three quarters of the respondents were male (77% Belgrade, 88% Nis). Most people who injected were aged 25 years or over. In Belgrade, 58% of the IDU population completed high school, compared to 76% in Nis. Over 75% of the IDU participants in Belgrade and Nis reported their employment status as unemployed.

Three multipliers were derived for Belgrade from the IBBS survey and these three questions on the survey were deliberately planned to match with relevant available benchmarks. The three multipliers were the proportion of people who had used needle exchange services, the proportion who had received HIV testing and finally the proportion who had undertaken detoxification treatment in the previous year.

The benchmark for the needle exchange multiplier was a central data base on data on numbers in receipt of needles. The remaining two benchmarks were the numbers of people who had untaken an HIV test and the number who had entered detoxification treatment in the period matching the multipliers.

For example, from the survey it was observed that 51% (0.51) of people aged 18 to 49 in Belgrade had received needle exchange services in the period 2009/10. This provided the multiplier. From the central database record system recording the number of people in receipt of needles in 2009/10 it was known that this number was 1654.

The estimate was then given as Total = 1654 × (1/0.51) = 3243. Details of the range prevalence estimates are provided in Table 2.5.

Discussion

This straightforward example illustrates how meaningful estimates can be produced for key planning discussions. Within this example a dedicated survey was devised to provide estimates of potential multipliers to be used with existing benchmarks. The benchmarks themselves provided some information on known numbers of cases engaged with service. Services knew they were not reaching all people who needed needle exchange or HIV testing or treatment. The survey carried out in the wider community with trained outreach workers provided access to a wider group

Table 2.5 Most at risk population—injecting drug users (IDU)

Most at risk population—injecting drug users (IDU)					
Location	Year	Age group	Prevalence estimate	95% C.I.	Method and definition of estimate
Belgrade	2009/2010	18–49	3243	[3121, 3376]	Multiplier ($m = 0.51$) from the 2009/10 IBBS on proportions reporting receiving needles in 2009 and benchmark ($n = 1654$) from 2010 needle exchange programmatic data
Belgrade	2009	18–49	4273	[3357, 5875]	Multiplier ($m = 0.11$) from the 2009/10 IBBS on proportions reporting receiving HIV testing in 2009 and benchmark ($m = 470$) from 2009 data on counts of individuals from the special hospital for drug use testing
Belgrade	2009	18–49	13,040	[10,867, 16,300]	Multiplier ($m = 0.10$) from the 2009/10 IBBS on proportions reporting receiving detoxification treatment in 2009 and benchmark ($n = 1304$) from 2009 counts of individuals receiving detoxification treatment

of people who injected drugs and from these people it could be seen what proportion had been in touch with these services. Once this proportion or multiplier was known, it could then be applied to the existing benchmark. This is a good example of how existing data can be useful and used as foundational building block for improved estimates of hidden prevalence.

However, estimates need to be interpreted cautiously given the methodological limitations. The sampling of people who injected drugs was not a random sample. This would not have been feasible. A snowball sample was used, people approached who were using drugs intravenously then recommended other people they knew who were using drugs intravenously and asked them to also complete the survey. As the people they know may also be attenders of the same services this can produce an overestimate of the multiplier and hence an underestimate of the prevalence.

Similarly benchmarks which came from existing data sources or databases and lists of people registered within the three services may not have been accurate. There was no audit of the accuracy of these benchmark lists, and they may have over counted or undercounted the number of people attending. Given these limitations it is wise to include confidence intervals on the estimates of the multipliers and the prevalence estimates to produce a range of potential minimum and maximum estimates.

To conclude, we can see within this case study how credible estimates can be achieved using both existing sources for a benchmark and a targeted survey with appropriate questions to provide relevant multipliers. This can result in preliminary estimates of the minimum and possible maximum size of the hidden population and can be of great benefit in aiding the planning and resourcing of services. Full details of this study can be found in Comiskey et al. (2013).

In our second case study, we explore the estimation of a child population, that is those children with a parent who uses substances and may need support.

Case Study 2.2: Estimating the Number of Children with a Parent Who Uses Substances Using the Multisource Enumeration Method

Introduction

Globally the potential impact of parental substance use on children has been documented. The effects are complex and can vary greatly, depending on both the drug, and the person. While there is probably no drug that is entirely harmless in all circumstances, it is important to accept that not all drug use is incompatible with being a good parent. Where adverse consequence for children do occur however, these are typically multiple and cumulative and will vary according to the child's stage of development. A review of these potential harms, in line with a child development framework has been provided at a European level by the EMCDDA (Comiskey, 2022). Within this guideline features of effective intervention programs have also been summarized given the available literature. However, before these programs can be implemented in a local community setting it is important to know how many children within that community are potentially in need of the intervention and external support. Within this case study we explore this challenge in a defined urban disadvantaged region of a major capital European city.

Methods

The multisource enumeration method with anonymous data was used for this challenge. As a unique identifier was not available for client's substance use services in the region an audit form for the collection of unique codes for each client within each service was developed. An example of this is provided in Tables 2.1, 2.2, 2.3, and 2.4. Each service completed the anonymous audit form either from their paper records or a database within their own individual service. The completed audit forms were then sent to a single person on the research team who oversaw the counting. This person then removed the duplicates that were found across services. For example, if someone was using an opiate agonist treatment service in one part of the community and a counselling service in another part of the community then this double counting of that person was recorded. This enabled the removal of duplicate counting of the same person across services.

Each service was asked to list if the person was a parent and if from their records, they could tell how any children that parent had. This had the limitation however that the child of both mother and a father could be counted twice. However, this may have been balanced by the omission of child information for some people who had not provided information on the number of children they may have had.

Results

A total of 14 local community agencies were asked to take part in the service audit, which also included qualitative questions and 79% of the agencies asked were able to participate. The remaining agencies were unable to participate due to annual leave, a lack of staff resources to provide the data, and/or a lack of available data on children.

Using the audit of the services and the removal of duplicates across the region, it was estimated that for the clients attending these services in 2014, there was a total of 751 children, this represented 3.7% of children in the area, at risk of being impacted by illicit drug use. This was a minimum estimate based on the multisource enumeration. It was found that for every one unique client identified in the region as using drugs, there was just under one child, with an exact ratio of 1 client to 0.88 children.

Discussion

This finding was very similar to the findings from the National Drug Treatment Outcome Research Study-ROSIE (Comiskey et al., 2009) in Ireland, which reported a figure of a ratio of 0.92 children to every one client in treatment for opiate use, and the Hidden Harm study in the UK, which found estimates reported of between 250,000 and 350,000 children of problem drug users in the UK—about one for every problem drug user. Details of these international estimates and this regional application of the method and the findings are provided by Galligan and Comiskey (2017) and Galligan and Comiskey (2019).

To conclude, several direct and indirect methods for estimating the hidden prevalence of substance use within a defined population, region, and time frame have been presented. From the simple multisource enumeration and multiplier methods to more sophisticated statistical modelling methods involving several indicators or data sources. The prevalence estimation method is continually evolving and drawing upon methods used in other disciplines from detailed mathematical disease modelling to engineering models to environmental modelling. One emerging approach which was originally developed to monitor the environmental impact of liquid household waste is wastewater monitoring. Wastewater analysis can be used to explore substance use within a city or region. It involves sampling a source of wastewater, such as a sewage influent to a wastewater treatment plant. This allows scientists to estimate the quantity of drugs consumed by a community by measuring the levels of illicit drugs and their metabolites excreted in urine. This novel application of the method has been piloted across a range of European cities (EMCDDA and Europol, 2023).

References

Allwright, S., Bradley, F., Long, J., Barry, J., Thornton, L., & Parry, J. V. (2000). Prevalence of antibodies to hepatitis B, hepatitis C, and HIV and risk factors in Irish prisoners: results of a national cross sectional survey. *Bmj, 321*(7253), 78–82.

Comiskey, C. M. (2001). Methods for estimating prevalence of opiate use as an aid to policy and planning. *Substance Use & Misuse, 36*(1–2), 131–150.

Comiskey, C. (2022). *Responses to the needs of children of people who use drugs*. Available at: https://www.emcdda.europa.eu/drugs-library/responses-needs-children-people-who-use-drugs_en. Accessed 04 June 2024.

Comiskey, C., Kelly, P., Leckey, Y., McCullough, L., O'Dúill, B., Stapleton, R., & White, E. (2009). *The ROSIE study: Drug treatment outcomes in Ireland.* Stationery Office.

Comiskey, C., Dempsey, O., Simic, D., & Baroš, S. (2013). Injecting drug users, sex workers and men who have sex with men: A national cross-sectional study to develop a framework and prevalence estimates for national HIV/AIDS programmes in the Republic of Serbia. *BMJ open, 3*(5), e002203.

Comiskey, C., Snel, A., & Banka, P. (2021). The second wave: Estimating the hidden asymptomatic prevalence of Covid-19 in Ireland as we plan for imminent immunisation. *HRB Open Research, 4*. https://doi.org/10.12688/HRBOPENRES.13206.2

EMCDDA. (2001). *Modelling drug use: methods to quantify and understand hidden processes* (92-9168-056-7). (EMCDDA Scientific Monograph Series No. 6 ISBN: 92-9168-056-7, Issue.

EMCDDA. (2002). *European network to develop policy relevant models and socio-economic analyses of drug use, consequences and interventions* Final report: Part 3 – Prevalence of drug use at the local level. Retrieved December 4, 2023, from https://www.emcdda.europa.eu/drugs-library/european-network-develop-policy-relevant-models-and-socio-economic-analyses-drug-use-consequences-and-interventions-final-report-part-3-%E2%80%93-prevalence-drug-use-local-level_en

EMCDDA. (2004). *Rapid assessment and response methods*. Retrieved November 28, 2023, from https://www.emcdda.europa.eu/drugs-library/rapid-assessment-and-response-methods_en

EMCDDA and Europol. (2023). *EU drug markets: In-depth analysis*. Retrieved August 28, 2023 from https://www.emcdda.europa.eu/publications/eu-drug-markets_en

ESPAD. (2019). *European school survey project on alcohol and other drugs*. Retrieved December 4, 2023, from http://www.espad.org/espad-report-2019

Galligan, K., & Comiskey, C. (2017). Estimating the number of children of parents who misuse substances, including alcohol across the communities of the Tallaght Drug and Alcohol Task Force (TDATF) region. Retrieved from https://www.drugsandalcohol.ie/29251/1/Estimating_the_number_of_children_ofparents_who-misuse-substances. pdf on, 24, 2021.

Galligan, K., & Comiskey, C. M. (2019). Hidden harms and the number of children whose parents misuse substances: A stepwise methodological framework for estimating prevalence. *Substance Use & Misuse, 54*(9), 1429–1437.

Golrokhi, R., Farhoudi, B., Taj, L., Pahlaviani, F. G., Mazaheri-Tehrani, E., Cossarizza, A., SeyedAlinaghi, S., Mohraz, M., & Voltarelli, F. A. (2018). HIV prevalence and correlations in prisons in different regions of the world: a review article. *The open AIDS journal, 12*, 81.

Hay, G., & Richardson, C. (2016). Estimating the prevalence of drug use using mark-recapture methods. *Statistical Science*, 191–204.

UNODC. (2003). *Estimating prevalence: Indirect methods for estimating the size of the drug problem.* Retrieved December 4, 2023 from https://www.unodc.org/documents/GAP/GAP%20Toolkit%20Module%202%20Final%20ENGLISH%2002-60052.pdf

Chapter 3
Addressing Needs: What Do Our Clients, Staff, and Community Need?

Setting the Scene

"I hope they give me Amanda's medication," said Tom. He was clearly anxious as he stood in the queue outside the dispensary window. "They're very strict here you know. If I ask for hers, they may not give me mine. Last week we were both here but one of the kids had a fever this morning and we couldn't send him to her sister who usually takes him. She has a new baby. We were hoping her mother could help us, but her emphysema is bad now, and she didn't want him in case she catches something."

Tom pulled hard on his cigarette; his hands were shaking as he closed his coat against the London morning cold. He nervously looked around. "Hell," replied Abram. "I wouldn't like to be in your shoes. Last week they almost didn't give me mine. I was five minutes late. Sabrina needed the car to bring the kids to dancing and I had to get the tube. I wish they had a creche or kids' room here … or at least give us a month's dose to take home. Don't they do that for other people on repeat meds? it would make life a lot easier." "Yeah, the least they could do is open the place for longer hours, even that would help." Tom hung his head, jittered and awaited his fate. The weed he had smoked last night to calm him seemed to have the opposite effect and he was worried about what might be in it.

Jen the pharmacist glanced resentfully down the length of the queue. It was the second time this week she had been asked to work overtime at short notice. Cutbacks and staff shortages were beginning to take their toll. They used to have a lovely community culture in this city treatment center but now everyone seemed stressed. They were also worried about anecdotal evidence on the rise in the number of recent fatalities and overdoses and wondered what was in these new synthetic cannabinoids being sold in the nearby streets…

C. Comiskey, *Addiction Research and Evaluation*, Advances in Mental Health and Addiction, https://doi.org/10.1007/978-3-031-65917-1_3

Introduction

Within the scenario above it can clearly be seen that the city center treatment clinic's clients and staff are under pressure and their needs are not being adequately addressed. Clients are stressed and worried about access, childcare, and the contents of their street drugs. Staff are over worked and concerned about the street drugs and funding cutbacks. The challenge for the clinic within this situation is to identify, prioritize, and address the varying needs given the resources available. Any solutions identified will also have to be adequately implemented to ensure they are operating as planned.

A needs analysis explores in a systematic way deficiencies and problems and identifies causes and solutions. Within a policy, service or individual personal treatment plan it can be considered as the process of identifying gaps between what should be provided and what is provided. Identifying and prioritizing conflicting needs is an ongoing challenge within policy, service delivery, and practice.

In the scenario above the needs of some individual clients accessing services in terms of childcare, opening hours and flexibility in prescribing practices are expressed. The needs of the pharmacy service in terms of staffing are also identified. However, the wider need of the community for access to drug testing facilities and the analysis the contents of local street drugs is also present.

The challenge is to identify the most pressing problem that can be realistically addressed within the national and local context. For example, within the scene above a dispensing clinic may not be able to provide drug testing facilities but they could easily provide warnings and harm reduction messages to each client as they attend. They may not be able to provide onsite childcare facilities as their premises or insurance may not be adequate. They may however seek to find funding for additional pharmacy staff and extend their opening hours. Similarly, without any large-scale direct costs they could consult with their stakeholders. They could decide to review their policy and the evidence available from the literature and other local substitution treatment services on repeat prescriptions. Extending the duration of the script for stable clients could possibly reduce the travel and childcare burden for the clients and at the same time assist with the staffing demands within the pharmacy service.

Key Principles When Responding to Needs

Any response to the needs of stakeholders must be conducted within the context of international, national, and local policies and frameworks. All of these will have an impact on the chosen approach and implementation of the change or intervention. Responses must also adhere to key principles, the first of these being:

- Respect for human rights, encompassing those of the clients, the staff, and the community within which they operate.

Further basic principles include:

- The right to access the highest attainable standards of physical and mental health.
- The right of people who use drugs and all relevant others to give informed consent to an intervention or treatment.
- The right to responses with ethical principles including confidentiality and ethical standards in the collection and storage of personal data.
- The right to equity of access to interventions.
- The right of access of service users and peer involvement in service design and delivery.
- Provision of responses that are appropriate for cultural and societal norms including cognizance of gender issues or other inequalities.
- Provision of properly designed responses based on needs and evidence informed, monitored, and evaluated on an appropriate basis.

According to the European Drugs Agency (EUDA) there are three broad stages for developing responses to drug problems and these are presented in Fig. 3.1.

Within this chapter, we focus on the problem definition stage which includes an assessment of needs. The needs assessment is guided by the European Drug Prevention Quality Standards (EDPQS) (EMCDDA, 2011). These standards focus on drug problems, but the principles can be applied to services and to practice.

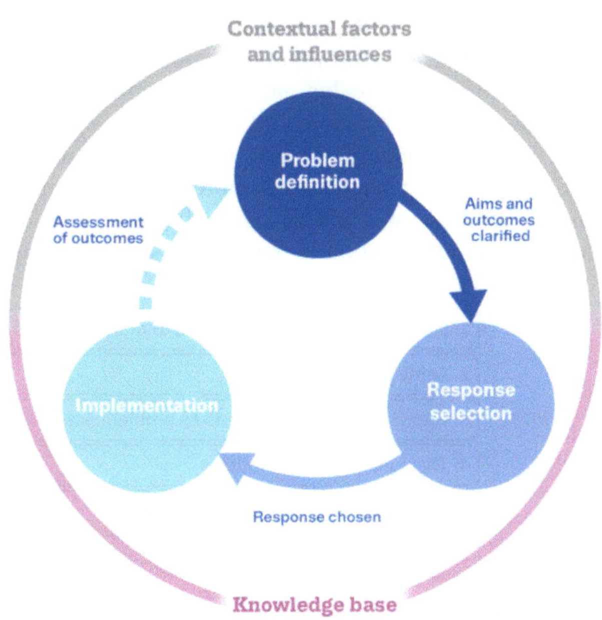

Fig. 3.1 The three broad stages of developing responses to drug problems. Courtesy of the EUDA. (Available from https://www.emcdda.europa.eu/publications/mini-guides/action-framework-for-developing-and-implementing-health-and-social-responses-to-drug-problems_e)

A Framework for Defining the Key Problem and Assessing Needs

Often as we have seen in our opening scenario there are seemingly competing needs between stakeholder groups. The pharmacist in our example needs fewer work hours, yet the clients need longer opening times. The center manager needs more resources, yet the budget has been cut back by local government. The first step is a recognition of the needs of the interrelated and possibly opposing groups. This is achieved by forming a stakeholder group given the stakeholder mapping exercise in Chap. 1. This group is tasked with defining the problem, overseeing the needs assessment, the identification of resources in terms both of facilitators and barriers and deciding on the most feasible response given the competing needs and the resources available. Figure 3.2 provides an overarching framework for this process.

Six Steps to Addressing Needs

The details for operationalizing each of the six steps within the framework are provided below.

1. Establish a stakeholder steering group with defined terms of reference.

A stakeholder group representing all those impacted by the problem and with access to resources to address it can be established. These terms of reference should include underlying values, decision-making mechanisms, reporting lines and governance, timing and duration of meetings, agenda setting, chairing, minute taking, and ultimate end date. Ensuring a common set of underlying values or philosophy is essential to reduce conflict and aid decision-making. How decisions are made is also important, for example, are decisions based on a voting mechanism? Or perhaps decisions can only be made if members are unanimous on a topic. This can be difficult to achieve in practice. A more pragmatic approach may be to base decision-making on consensus. Not all may be happy with a decision, but they are willing to compromise for the good of the steering committee and the goal of addressing the

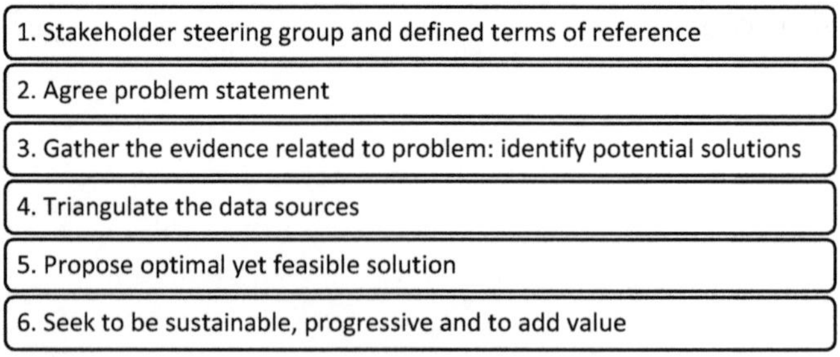

Fig. 3.2 The six steps framework for defining and addressing a problem

needs. Draft terms of reference with an outline of key principles can be prepared by the hosting organization and sent to the stakeholders in advance of the first meeting. Ensuring them that the draft is open to change and is merely drafted to facilitate the first meeting and save time within the meeting for constructive discussion.

2. Agree the problem statement.

It is important that a concise, clear, and succinct problem statement is agreed by the steering committee. In our setting the scene example the problem may be stated as,

"The pharmacy service is not meeting the needs of our clients and our staff. Within the past week all pharmacy staff have been asked to work overtime at short notice and the service has received verbal and written complaints from clients. Given our recent growth in client numbers this service is no longer fit for purpose."

The problem statement helps the steering committee stay focused on the key challenge. It will also help with communicating the challenge to others. It serves as the basis for developing a plan and gathering the appropriate data to begin to solve the problem.

3. Gather the background evidence and data related to the problem and potential solutions.

To understand the problem and consider solutions background evidence and data needs to be gathered from a range of sources and stakeholders. Evidence in the form of published findings from other studies can be sought to provide examples from best international practice and standards relating to the challenge. Many international guidelines based on peer reviewed studies are available online. The United Nations Office for Drugs and Crime (UNODC) provide global advice on a range of drug issues (see https://www.unodc.org/). Within the United States, the Substance Abuse and Mental Health Services Administration (SAMHSA) provides a wealth of relevant resources (see https://www.samhsa.gov/). Within the European Union and neighboring countries, the European Drugs Agency (EUDA) formerly known as the European Monitoring Centre for Drugs and Drug Addiction (EMCDDA) also provides a range of best practice guidelines (see https://www.emcdda.europa.eu/index_en).

In terms of evidence from data, there are two basic types of data, quantitative and qualitative. Quantitative data can be measured on a numerical scale and can be analyzed using statistical methods and displayed using tables and graphs. Qualitative data are not intended to be measured or counted rather they relate to the quality or character of something. They provide an understanding of social situations and of people's experiences. They are generally expressed in words, pictures, and objects and are collected in qualitative methods such as interviews, observations, focus groups or visuals.

If some resources are available new data can be generated (this is called primary data) or if resources are very limited existing quantitative and/or qualitative data can be used (this is known as secondary data). Data can be objective; it can be an objective measurement or an objective analysis of existing records or documents. Data can also be subjective, for example recording of individual peoples' experiences or opinions.

In our pharmacy example it would be good to capture a range of data sources. The pharmacy service might do an audit, that is, an objective analysis of the changes in the numbers of clients registered within the past 12 months and the compare this with the opening times of the service within the past 12 months. The center manger might do an audit of existing staffing and recorded working hours. These two exercises would provide some objective secondary data.

To seek opinions on solutions to the challenge the pharmacy could also generate some new primary data. They could do an anonymous survey of their clients asking them to rank their preferences for a range of potential pharmacy improvements. Alternatively, instead of the service suggesting potential improvements they might work with their service users and staff within focus groups to share their experiences and needs. Given these they could then co-design potential solutions for presentation to the stakeholder steering group.

4. Triangulate the gathered data sources.

Hales et al. (2010) provide an excellent introduction to triangulation explaining that while it originally arose within mathematics as a means of locating a point on a triangle it extended to Global Positioning Systems (GPS) to locate a place given information from usually four satellites. It is now used within research to improve the analysis and interpretation of findings from various types of studies. While there can be different types of triangulations, the triangulation within our needs analysis is a triangulation of the data.

Data triangulation is, "the use of a variety of data sources including time, space, and persons, in a study. Findings can be corroborated and any weaknesses in the data can be compensated for by the strengths of other data, thereby increasing the validity and reliability of the results. The approach has been used in many sectors to strengthen conclusions about findings and to reduce the risk of false interpretations" (UNAIDS, 2010:14).

A larger pool of relevant data sources enables areas of convergence and divergence to be discovered that may not have been identified or noticed in the data from a single source. It is within these convergences and divergences that the key findings and recommendations will emerge.

To undertake a triangulation of the varying data sources the goal or objective of the triangulation must be agreed. This should reflect the problem statement. The data then needs to be collated and aggregated as appropriate given the data type. Key findings from the data sources need to be summarized and presented. The next step is to then analyze and draw collective conclusions from the data related to the problem solution.

5. Propose an optimal yet feasible solution.

When drawing conclusions and recommendations from the data triangulation, the team should be looking for convergence in findings across the data sources. Convergent findings will point in the direction of an optimal solution for the problem given the input from the varying data sources and stakeholders. This convergence will add strength to the conclusions and recommendations. Similarly, divergence in findings needs to be considered and explained. It is important to consider if this divergence highlights perhaps a potential problem with implementing the proposed solution. For example, does the divergence take away from the feasibility of the proposed solution? Enablers and barriers to implementation of a new practice or policy change is discussed in detail in Chap. 10.

6. Seek to be sustainable, progressive, and to add value.

Finally, when the stakeholder steering group proposes a solution it should aim to be sustainable in terms of resources needed and used. It should also seek to add value to exiting resources and services rather than taking away from resources needed elsewhere. A question to ask is, "Does the solution add value to the service in some way or are there any unforeseen consequences?" It is important that the proposed solution obtains input and consensus from each of the representative stakeholder groups. Finally, a solution should seek to be progressive and an exemplar of best practice that can be piloted initially and then mainstreamed and disseminated once it has been proven within the context of the setting.

Two case studies illustrating these steps are provided.

Case Study 3.1: The Challenge of Identifying the Needs of Homeless People in Substance Use Recovery

Introduction

The United Nations (UN) Housing Unit provided a range of definitions and some pre-COVID-19 global statistics on homelessness. According to the UN, homelessness is one of the most acute forms of material deprivation. It refers to the inability of people to enjoy permanent accommodation. Homelessness can include street homelessness and rough sleepers, people staying in housing with inadequate, unsafe conditions, people living in temporary or emergency accommodation such as tents, dormitories, or hotel rooms and finally people enduring hidden homelessness who may be sleeping on a friend or family members couch or floor space.

As of June 2019, it was estimated that 1.6 billion people worldwide lived in inadequate housing conditions and people experiencing street homelessness face negative outcomes related to mortality, health, ability to earn a basic income and other basic elements of survival (Salcedo, 2019). In terms of health and well-being it is recognized that among people who use drugs and who experience homelessness there are intersecting social, mental, and physical health risks that significantly increase morbidity and mortality (EMCDDA, 2023). The World Health Organization provides an illustration of these additional challenges visually with the work of one nurse working with homeless people who use substances and are hospitalized (WHO, 2020).

In terms of people using substances, within one city center homeless service, a residential treatment service for those who have exited a clinical detoxification program is provided. The service is offered over three stages. Stage 1 facilitates the very early stages of recovery and provides 24-h on-site support. Stage 2 sees a reduction in the 24/7 on-site support and an escalation of community engagement. Stage 3 is the final phase of the recovery service and provides visiting support to the housing. Clients at this stage usually access aftercare services in preparation for their move to independent living. The housing organization wanted to explore the challenge of addressing the needs across the three-stage recovery pathway from the perception of the wider governance structures, the leadership team, the staff, and those in the recovery accommodation.

Methods

A small stakeholder group to support the research process and guide the researchers was established by the homeless organization. Prior to any research being conducted a protocol for the study design was developed which included an agreed problem statement expressed in the form of the study aim. This was expanded upon by developing a set of study objectives that would help realize the aim and address the problem statement. The organization recognized that their key problem was the challenges in the recovery pathway faced by both people who used their services and their staff and they wished to assess the needs of their staff and clients.

To gather the background evidence and data related to the problem and potential solutions, a range of primary and secondary, quantitative, and qualitative, primary and secondary data sources were assessed. A mixed methods design was chosen as the most suitable approach. This approach was applied to bring the strengths of both quantitative and qualitative research together to compare and confirm the findings across multiple sets of data in a final data triangulation stage.

A retrospective analysis was conducted of client records using existing secondary datasets. A prospective measurement of the processes and impact of the recovery journey (post detoxification) from the service users' perspective using the validated surveys, the Opiate Treatment Index; the General Health Questionnaire, a Post-Traumatic Stress Disorder Scale, the Adverse Childhood Experience scale, and the Journey Travelled Tool was used. One-to-one interviews to investigate the enablers and barriers to a successful completion of stages 1, 2, and 3 of the recovery as perceived by staff, and leadership were conducted. Finally, a documentary analysis reviewing, the policies, management, and leadership gaps was also conducted.

Results

The retrospective data available in the organization was impressive, however further quality improvements were required to ensure data accuracy. The prospective quantitative findings on clients who were recruited at baseline and followed up 6 months later showed that there was a reduction in the number of overall general health problems reported. Psychological well-being did not significantly change between baseline and follow-up; however, those recruited within stage 2 showed a marked improvement.

There was a larger than expected change in anxiety symptoms within those recruited in stage 3, the final stage of the recovery journey. A possible explanation for this change may have been due to increased anxiety levels of participants on monthly residency contracts. At this stage of their recovery pathway clients were expected to move out of their existing accommodation and into independent housing.

The results also showed a marked improvement in self-confidence, goal setting, and self-efficacy across all three groups, however, individuals' confidence in their literacy and communications skills appeared to be quite low.

In terms of findings from the qualitative interviews, several areas for attention were identified including the alignment of the specific recovery strategy to the overarching strategy of the homeless organization. The complexity of the recovery service had also outgrown the current systems which had supported the service delivery, and the structure was resettling following some changes.

From a leadership style point of view, the difficulties in staff retention and recruitment and the administration burden of regulation were dictating the leadership style with managers coping with urgent rather than important demands.

Discussion

The triangulation of the multilevel data findings provided a holistic picture of current and future optimal service delivery needs from the perspective of service users, service providers, and organizational leadership. These were proposed as a set of optimal sustainable recommendations to the problem as summarized in Table 3.1.

Table 3.1 Summary of set of optimal sustainable recommended solutions for a homeless service following a needs analysis with data triangulation

Current needs	Area of need	Potential recommended solution
Communicate the current strategy of the community reinforcement approach (CRA) to all team members on recruitment and induction. Ensure consistency in language	**Strategy**	Develop a strategy for the treatment service which is consultative and participatory and reflects short–/ medium-term objectives
Communicate the structure, purpose, and responsibilities of team members clearly which will improve team cohesion and cooperation. Ensure consistency of message and terminology i.e., key worker, project worker, support worker	**Structure**	Ensure that changes in structure are in line with the long-term strategy of the service and are consistent with sector terminology and expectations
Document and communicate a client flow through process which is flexible yet consistent and transparent. This will require additional staff training and senior commitment to the process, including the monitoring and management of data from the new database system	**Systems**	Ensure that the new data collection process is delivery focused and data is useful, usable, and current. This will inform the systems, structures, and future strategies of the service Ensure that data captured is suitable for mapping relevant long-term outcomes at the individual level. These may include physical, mental, and social functioning needs at baseline and at regular follow-up points. This being at initial assessment and at exist at a minimum
The leadership style is viewed as supportive, but support must be provided for leadership to retain their skills and experience into the future	**Styles**	Develop a pipeline of leadership from within the team and develop a consistent leadership development program
The greatest asset of the organization is the team members, the organization should capitalize on the excellence through people award and continue to develop their peer-to-peer policy on recruitment	**Staff**	Develop a publishable career pathway for peer-to-peer recovery team members
Ensure all training is up to date on CRA and that team members understand ethos of approach and its place in the recovery journey. Incorporate trauma training in standard staff training	**Skills**	Future-proof skills set of teams to provide cutting-edge alternative therapy which is innovative and services the needs of a changing client. Ensure all practices are trauma informed
Document the shared values of the recovery services including the successes and the ethos of the CRA so it forms a solid foundation on which to build the service	**Shared values**	Ensure that the organization remains a "community" internally and externally which includes and celebrates the addiction and recovery service

Case Study 3.2: The Challenge of Identifying the Needs of People Accessing Integrated Alcohol Treatment Services

Introduction

In 2019, an analysis of the global burden of 87 risk factors in 204 countries found that alcohol use was the leading risk factor for attributable burden of disease among people aged 25–49 years and the second leading risk factor among those aged from 10 to 24 years. Taking all burdens into account, globally alcohol was the ninth-leading risk factor among all ages (GBD 2019 Risk Factors Collaborators, 2020).

Furthermore, it has been demonstrated that despite making up only 25% of the population, hazardous and harmful drinkers accounted for 78% of alcohol consumption and 68% of alcohol revenue within England (Bhattacharya et al., 2018) and similar statistics have been cited for the United States (Cook, 2011). These proportions of sales reflect what is known as *The Pareto Principle* which states that "the top 20 percent of buyers for any consumer product account for fully 80 percent of sales," (Cook, 2011). Given the level of burden of alcohol use the range of health and social issues impacting upon people who experience harmful drinking are considerable.

Integrated health was developed to address fragmented health and social care needs and provide services for individuals with complex healthcare issues. Definition of integrated healthcare have varied depending on the perspective of the person, the service or the system. This has been addressed by the International Foundation for Integrated Care (Lennox-Chhugani et al., 2022) who recognize a continuum of definitions of integrated care. This continuum can equally have a narrow definition at one end and a broader definition at the other end. At the narrow end it includes initiatives seeking to improve outcomes of care by overcoming issues of fragmentation through linkage or coordination of services along the continuum of care within a health system. At the broader end of the continuum, integrated care has been defined as a system that addresses fragmentation beyond the boundaries of the formal health and care system, understanding well-being in terms of quality of life and referring to people's capacity to live a healthy, meaningful, creative, and fulfilling life (Lennox-Chhugani et al., 2022).

Within a national healthcare service, two pilot services were developed to provide integrated alcohol services to people experiencing harmful alcohol use. A community-based team delivered evidence-based psychosocial interventions and family support and developed integrated care pathways. This team was integrated with a liaison nurse based in the acute hospital setting.

The two pilot services developed separately and the problem for the national funders was a lack of evidence supporting the models of care provided, the processes of integration and the impact of the pilot service on the outcomes and care for the person. It was decided to establish a wide national steering group representing a range of stakeholders representing the partners needed for the integration of key services and a smaller project support group to address the challenge. The problem statement could be stated as: "Two pilot integrated alcohol services have been developed, yet we have no information on what is working, what are the barriers and enablers and how the service can be scaled up and sustainably rolled out nationally."

Methods

An initial international literature review exploring the design and integration of alcohol services was conducted. A narrative synthesis of findings on what worked was prepared summarizing the evidence or lack thereof for a range of service design features (McCarthy et al., 2022).

To gather the background evidence related to the national problem a concurrent, qualitative dominant, mixed methods design was implemented (C. Comiskey et al., 2023). People who used alcohol-related services and their families, friends, and supporters were invited to participate in an online survey. Additional open-ended questions seeking feedback were also asked of families, friends, and others. One-to-one semi-structured interviews were conducted with people who used the piloted alcohol services and people who provide these services. Ethical approval was also sought and granted.

Simple descriptive statistics were prepared from the online surveys. An inductive thematic analysis as detailed by Braun and Clarke (2006) informed by the People First Framework of Comiskey (2019) was prepared for the qualitative interviews. Word clouds were also used to summarize service users' comments on enablers and barriers to accessing services. A triangulation of findings from both aspects of the study was conducted to identify areas of convergence and divergence across the participants. A visual spider graph was used to represent the key themes as identified from each participating group.

Results

The qualitative interviews with service users ($n = 10$) were brief and had an average duration of 16 min. In terms of referrals to the services, 20% of participants had been referred by a family member or friend, 10% by an employer, 10% by court services and the majority, 60% ($n = 6$) had been referred by their GP or hospital nurse. Of those who had accessed the service, 70% had previously accessed and tried several services in the past. Of those who had previously accessed supports or services, several services or a combination of services had been explored with a view to reducing or quitting problem alcohol consumption.

While the levels of satisfaction with the service received was 100% across all service users interviewed, satisfaction with counselling services was most frequently mentioned. An analysis of enablers across the most frequently mentioned

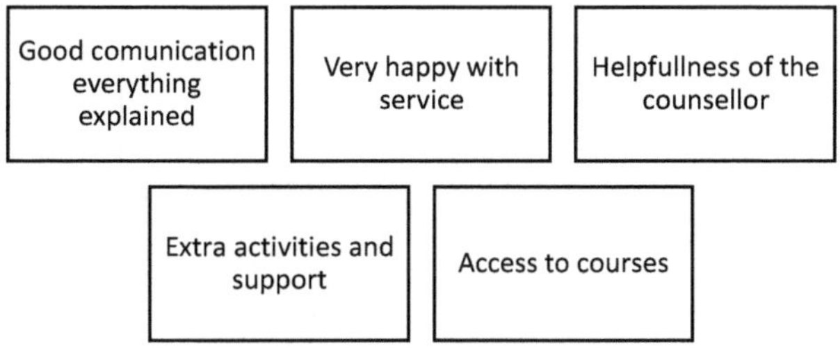
Good comunication everything explained
Very happy with service
Helpfullness of the counsellor
Extra activities and support
Access to courses

Fig. 3.3 Most frequently mentioned enablers identified in an assessment of client's needs in an integrated alcohol service

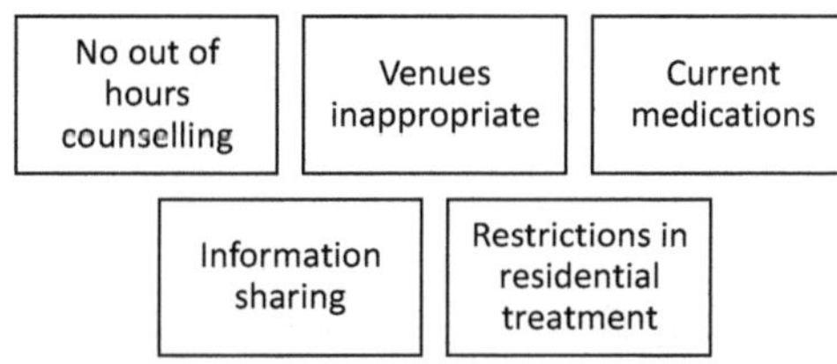

Fig. 3.4 Most frequently mentioned barriers identified in an assessment of client's needs in an integrated alcohol service

services particularly noted good communications, access to extra supports such as funding, support activities, and educational courses. This is demonstrated in Fig. 3.3.

The potential barriers to accessing services as advised by the service users are listed below in order of frequency of mentions. These are displayed in Fig. 3.4.

The most frequently mentioned barrier to accessing the integrated service was the degree of flexibility offered by counselling services. Several participants felt that if they were not self-employed or unemployed, they would not be able to confidentially attend the counselling services, which were mainly scheduled during working hours, 9 am–5 pm, Monday to Friday. This barrier was important for the rollout and scale up of accessible and sustainable integrated services.

Twelve interviews were conducted with service providers. Providers were based in a wide range of addiction services, including primary care, hospitals, community care, and residential care. They included general practitioners, nurses, addiction counsellors, case managers, and service managers. Three general themes emerged from the analysis, these were standard operating procedures and structures, services meeting clients' needs, and addressing the bigger picture.

Service user's family, friends, and supporters provided written responses to several open-ended questions on alcohol treatment services in general. Sixteen people provided responses and indicated that the half of the service users had accessed both inpatient and outpatient services. Ease of access was regarded as difficult or very difficult by 44% of respondents. Exploring the barriers, the reasons cited were, hard to navigate (29%), lack of information (14%), lack of support (21%), lack of resources (75%), and duration of wait (29%). The themes extracted from the family, friends, and supporters of the service user were concerned with two areas. These were, firstly, increased awareness and community education, including early interventions and detection and secondly, increased staff training.

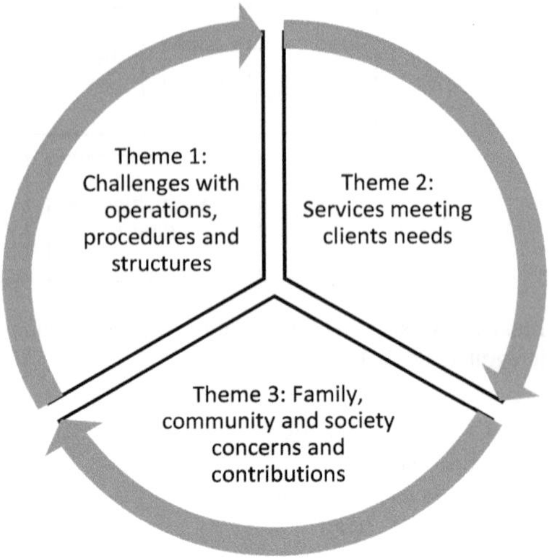

Fig. 3.5 A triangulation of convergent findings from all three stakeholder groups

A triangulation of convergent findings from all three stakeholder groups is provided in Fig. 3.5. We can see from this figure the importance of theme 1 on standard operating procedures. The importance of theme 2, particularly accessibility of the service including addressing the criteria for service provision. Finally, public health supporting families of service users with early interventions and detection.

Discussion

The literature review on effective services combined with the triangulation of findings provided the supporting international and local evidence to inform recommendations for solutions to the problem statement.

To address the lack of standardization in the model of integrated care within the piloted alcohol services, the development of a manualized program with shared and standardized assessments was proposed.

To address accessibility a hybrid model of care with face to face and an online or telecare system for after-hours delivery was suggested. The evidence for the efficacy of online-only services was weak, according to McCarthy et al. (2022), but the evidence for hybrid models was stronger. Once the hybrid model was developed in partnership with all stakeholders then the development of the manual with the inclusion of appropriate outcome measurements could be initiated.

To address education and training it was recommended that once the online system and manual was developed a hybrid model for continuing professional development could also be developed. This would address the training on the standard operating procedures related to the model of care and related topics. This hybrid manual could continue to develop and be built upon to include information for families, friends, and supporters. The need for ongoing training and support for all stakeholders was clearly stated in the review by McCarthy et al. (2022).

To conclude the combination of the background international literature review and the local stakeholder evidence provided a thorough description of the needs of the integrated alcohol service and how best given the international evidence they could be addressed to provide a sustainable solution and allow the scale up and roll out of a service that met the needs of all concerned.

References

Bhattacharya, A., Angus, C., Pryce, R., Holmes, J., Brennan, A., & Meier, P. S. (2018). How dependent is the alcohol industry on heavy drinking in England? *Addiction, 113*(12), 2225–2232.

Braun, V., & Clarke, V. (2006). Using thematic analysis in psychology. *Qualitative Research in Psychology, 3*(2), 77–101. https://doi.org/10.1191/1478088706qp063oa

Comiskey, C. (2019). Addiction Debates: *Hot Topics from Policy to Practice*. SAGE. United Kingdom. https://us.sagepub.com/enus/nam/addiction-debates/book269028I SBN9781526495761

Comiskey, C., Kelly, P., Hennessy, A., Hyland, M., O'Neill, D., Banka Cullen, S., & Lavelle Cafferky, S. (2023). *A consultation to inform the delivery of new integrated alcohol services*.

Cook, P. J. (2011). *Paying the tab: The costs and benefits of alcohol control*. Princeton University Press. http://www.jstor.org/stable/j.ctt7shzt

EMCDDA. (2011). *European drug prevention quality standards (EDPQS)*. Retrieved October 9, 2023, from https://www.emcdda.europa.eu/publications/manuals/prevention-standards_en

EMCDDA. (2023). *Homelessness and drugs: health and social responses*. Retrieved October 17, 2023, from https://www.emcdda.europa.eu/publications/mini-guides/homelessness-and-drugs-health-and-social-responses_en

GBD 2019 Risk Factors Collaborators. (2020). Global burden of 87 risk factors in 204 countries and territories, 1990–2019: A systematic analysis for the Global Burden of Disease Study 2019. *396*, 1223–1249. https://doi.org/10.1016/S0140-6736(20)30752-2.

Hales, D., Peersman, G., Rugg, D., & Kiwango, E. (2010). An introduction to triangulation. In *UNAIDS, joint UN Programme HIV/AIDS*. https://www.unaids.org/sites/default/files/sub_landing/files/10_4-Intro-to-triangulation-MEF.pdf

Lennox-Chhugani, N., Alvarez-Rosete, A., Aldasoro, E., & Gil-Salmeron, A. (2022). Promoting integrated care across the world: IFIC Annual Survey 2022.

McCarthy, E., Prakashini Banka, S., Eustace-Cook, J., Tobin, K., & Comiskey, C. (2022). *An evidence review on effective interventions and approaches in the delivery of integrated alcohol Services in Community*. Lisbon Addictions 2022. https://www.lisbonaddictions.eu/lisbon-addictions-2022/presentations/literature-review-using-systematic-approach-effective-interventions-and-approaches

Salcedo. (2019). *HOMELESSNESS & THE SDGs*. Retrieved October 17, 2023, from https://www.un.org/development/desa/dspd/wpcontent/uploads/sites/22/2019/07/SALCEDO_Jesus_Presentation_2-1.pdf

UNAIDS. (2010). *An Introduction to Triangulation*, UNAIDS 20, AVENUE APPIA, CH-1211 GENEVA 27, SWITZERLAND. Retrieved October 17, 2023, from https://www.unaids.org/sites/default/files/sub_landing/files/10_4-Intro-to-triangulation-MEF.pdf

World Health Organization. (2020). *Nursing homeless people in Ireland*. Retrieved October 17, 2023, from Nursing homeless people in Ireland (who.int).

Chapter 4
Prevention and Intervention: What Are the Components of Successful Interventions?

Setting the Scene

Kim stood with her back to the kitchen facing the sink. She had found with her two children that it was usually more productive of open conversation if she didn't look at them directly as they addressed challenging topics. This time however the shoe was on the other foot. Ari, her daughter was explaining how difficult it was to refuse a drink when it was offered to you by your boss especially after the hugely successful completion of an event.

"I didn't like to refuse the glass of champagne they offered," said Ari. "They were all in high spirits and if you're the one not drinking it sets you apart as a kill joy. They were all older than me, so I didn't like to tell them I don't drink. I just accepted it to be sociable. I thought I could sip it. But then they ordered a full bottle of expensive red wine and poured me a glass of that too. At that stage it was too late to tell them I didn't drink! They would think me weird especially as I had said nothing previously."

Ari was clearly upset and frustrated. Guiltily Kim recalled the numerous times that they as a family had opened a bottle of champagne to celebrate and had repeatedly asked Ari if she would like to try some even though they knew she didn't drink. Kim had never thought about how family or other peer pressures may have impacted her teenage children. She felt ashamed that she as the parent hadn't appreciated this.

Kim was also proud but a little sad that Ari had to face similar pressure from her work colleagues and her boss. Her personal shame strengthened her resolve to try harder in future. The irony of this wasn't lost on her given she was a teacher and had been responsible for rolling out prevention programs among teenagers in her school.

C. Comiskey, *Addiction Research and Evaluation*, Advances in Mental Health and Addiction, https://doi.org/10.1007/978-3-031-65917-1_4

Introduction

The youth response to the World Drug Report (WDR) 2023 (Paradigma Youth Coalition, 2023) commends the WRD for their focus on youth and on prevention. They highlight the challenges faced by youth in not only accessing services but also in receiving appropriate drug prevention education that enables them to make informed, harm reducing choices. Examples of the need for this can be found globally and in increasingly diverse settings. Within South Korea it has been reported that young affluent school goers were deliberately targeted with free drinks they were told would help them concentrate during their exams. The drinks were laced with methamphetamine and ecstasy. Their parents were subsequently blackmailed for money to prevent the perpetrators reporting their drugged children to authorities (CAST, 2023).

Within India, Pattojoshi and Tikka (2020) have explored school-based substance use and prevention within Indian schools. Authors noted that both street children and school going students have been found to use various substances. Among children living on the streets, prevalence rates as high as 83% have been reported. However, among school goers, almost one in five are also affected by substance use. Clearly all children need support and varying pathways to access appropriate prevention and treatment programs are essential for the varying settings. Community, work place, and school-based settings have been targeted within India to address the challenges they are facing (Malick, 2018; Pattojoshi & Tikka, 2020).

The World Drug Report of 2023 produced a special points of interest booklet (UNODC, 2023b). Within this booklet, four key messages of equal priority were highlighted. One, it was noted that world drug-related challenges are hindering the progress of the Sustainable Development Goals. Two, law enforcement responses need to keep pace with agile criminal business models. Three, public health must remain the priority in the context of developing drug control regulation and more must be invested in research to monitor the effects of policies. The fourth key message having equal priority with the other three messages was the statement that the need for prevention and access to evidence-informed treatment must be increased otherwise drug-related challenges will leave more people behind. Given the current global inequitable access to treatment services the need for prevention is of the utmost importance.

Reducing these inequalities in prevention and treatment access among vulnerable and marginalized groups is critical according to UNODC (2023b) and this is reflected in the global examples discussed. While higher socioeconomic groups are more likely to initiate drug use, lower socioeconomic groups are more likely to suffer from drug use disorders. The demand for treating such disorders is largely unmet and large disparities in access exist. Only one in five people who needed treatment receive it and not all treatment provided respects human rights and is based on scientific evidence.

Young people are the most vulnerable to using drugs and disparities within them exist. For example, within Africa, 70% of people receiving drug treatment are below the age of 35. Possible responses to these challenges according to the UNODC (2023b) are large-scale drug use prevention initiatives that are within school, family, and community settings. These are needed to address both the rise in drug use disorders and the rise in mental health conditions. These two conditions we know are linked, and one challenge can exacerbate the other. This comorbidity of challenges will be addressed in more detail in Chap. 5 where we discuss treatment and comorbidity respectively. Within this chapter the challenge of evidence-based prevention is addressed.

Defining Prevention

Within broader healthcare prevention the natural history of a disease is grouped into five stages, these are underlying, susceptible, subclinical, clinical, and finally recovery, disability or death. Preventative health has developed to reflect these stages of a disease. The stages of prevention are primordial prevention, primary prevention, secondary prevention, and tertiary prevention.

Primordial prevention targets the underlying stage of a natural disease by targeting the underlying social conditions that promote disease onset. Prevention measures are usually delivered through policy and laws. An example might be a sugar tax to prevent obesity in children (Kisling & Das, 2023). Primary prevention is targeted at susceptible populations or individuals. Secondary prevention targets seemingly healthy individuals who have subclinical forms of the disease. Tertiary prevention targets people with symptoms and aims to reduce the severity of the disease.

Finally quaternary prevention, which has been redefined in recent years, is actions taken to identify patients at risk of over medicalization, to protect such patients from new medical conditions and to suggest to the patient other interventions which are ethical. According to Martins et al. (2018, p. 107), this definition has been modified and is now defined as, "an action taken to protect individuals (persons/patients) from medical interventions that are likely to cause more harm than good."

Within substance use, prevention is considered one part of a continuum of what is known as behavioral health. The other parts are health promotion, treatment, and recovery. This continuum could be said to reflect the continuum seen within disease progression. Each aspect of the continuum is important, promotion supports positive behaviors, prevention reduces risk, treatment is for those with a diagnosed substance use disorder, and recovery helps people define what they wish to prioritize as important to them after treatment (Prevention Action Alliance, 2023).

The prevention approaches for substance use and related issues also mirror disease prevention models. According to the EMCDDA and Europol (2023), environmental prevention, similar to primordial prevention, aims to change cultural, physical, and economic environments within which people make behavioral choices to use substances. Such prevention strategies at this level may include bans on tobacco use in public spaces or minimum unit pricing on alcohol products.

Universal prevention, like primary prevention addresses entire populations usually in school, community, or work settings. Prevention at this stage within these settings aims to give people the social competence to avoid or delay the initiation of substance use. Selective prevention intervenes with specific groups, perhaps communities or families who are more likely to develop substance use disorders. Finally, according to the Prevention Action Alliance (2023), indicated prevention helps people who are vulnerable to substance use disorder. For example, it may help students who have shown signs of substance use but do not have a diagnosed disorder.

In summary we have then, environmental, universal, selective, and indicated prevention.

Developmental Approach to Prevention

In addition to the prevention approaches, UNODC and WHO (UNODC, 2023a; WHO, 2018) in their international standards for drug prevention interventions and policies, highlight that it is essential to take a childhood developmental approach. Within the standards, they focus on the prevention of drug use initiation and the prevention of transition to drug use disorders. The standards do not address secondary and tertiary prevention interventions, such as treatment of drug use disorders and the prevention of health and social consequences of drug use and drug use disorders. Similarly, they do not address law enforcement efforts for drug control. They do however address primary or universal prevention and selected prevention for certain groups. As a developmental approach is taken the standards are presented according to the child or adult stage. This is presented in Table 4.1.

Table 4.1 The age-related developmental stages for prevention interventions

Pregnancy
Infancy (under 2 years of age)
Early childhood (2–5 years old)
Middle childhood (primary school age, 6–10 years old approximately)
Early adolescent (middle school/junior high school, 11–14 years old)
Adolescent (senior high school, late teens from 15–18 or 19 years of age)
Adulthood (all subsequent years)
This can be further classified as, young adulthood for 20- to 25-year-olds during the college or university years and all adults over 25 years

Risk and Protective Factors for Prevention

Like other behavioral issues, substance use has been identified by prevention scientists as a developmental issue which varies by the age of the child, young person, or adult (EMCDDA, 2019). The risk and protective factors begin early and in general these behaviors occur in late childhood and adolescence. This requires an understanding of the prevention needs at different ages, starting with infants and very young children, progressing through the more vulnerable teenage and young adult years, and continuing throughout adulthood. Age-appropriate intervention strategies addressing the risk and protective factors across the lifespan are important (WHO, 2018).

As with many health conditions, everyone is susceptible to addiction but there are certain recognized risk and protective factors that can increase or decrease a person's likelihood of developing an addiction to substances. These factors can be divided into two broad categories. According to NIDA (2012), these can be either environmental or biological. Environmental can include a person's home, family, peers, school, and community setting. Biological can include a person's gender, genetics, and mental disorder.

According to NIDA (2021), it is estimated that genetics account for between 40% and 60% of a person's risk of addiction. Research on environmental and biological risk and protective factors is continually advancing. A recent systematic review of individual, family, and community factors by Nawi et al. (2021) provided a summary. However, it must be stressed that the list provided below in Table 4.2 is not exhaustive.

Given the breath of risk and protective factors Nawi et al. (2021) highlight that prevention programs will need to be designed to be extensive and reflect the varying levels of individual, family, and community.

The key components required within prevention are addressed in the following sections.

Underlying Theory of Change and Related Logic Models

When rolling out any intervention or prevention program it is important to ask, "Why do we expect this change in behavior to happen as a result of this intervention?" The answer to this question is provided by the theory underlying the program or the intervention. According to the Center for Effective Services, CES (2022),

> *A Theory of Change is an explicit, step-by-step statement of the expected relationship between the intervention and the outcome. It outlines how what we put in (input X) allows to do something (output Y), leading to a change in circumstance (outcome Z). The inputs, outputs and outcomes should be conceptually and practically linked, including what evidence we have that it will work.*

Table 4.2 A compilation of risk and protective factors at the individual, family, and community levels as identified by Nawi et al. (2021), Prevention Action Alliance (2023) and NIDA (2021)

Risk factors: individual	Protective factors: individual
Traits of high impulsivity	Individual traits of optimism
Rebelliousness	High level of mindfulness
Emotional regulation impairment	Having social phobia
Low religious	Having strong beliefs against substance abuse
Pain catastrophic	Desire to maintain one's health
Homework completeness	High paternal awareness of drug abuse
Total screen time and alexithymia	School connectedness
Experience of maltreatment or a negative upbringing	Structured activity
Having psychiatric disorders such as conduct problems and major depressive disorder	Having strong religious beliefs
Previous e-cigarette exposure	Good self-control
Behavioral addiction	
Low-perceived risk	
High-perceived drug accessibility	
High-attitude to use synthetic drugs	
Risk factors: family	**Protective factors: family**
Prenatal maternal smoking	Positive relationship
Poor maternal psychological control	Parental monitoring and support
Low parental education	
Negligence	
Poor supervision	
Uncontrolled pocket money	
Presence of substance-using family members	
Parents or older family members who use drugs or misuse alcohol, or who break the law	
Risk factors: community	**Protective factors: community**
Having peers who abuse drugs	Anti-drug policies at school
Community poverty	Neighborhood resources
Struggling in school	
Poor social skills	

When developing a theory of change it is important to think of a series of what the CES call a series of "if, then" relationships. If we do this action, then this action will happen. Each "if, then" relationship should be based on previous information, research, or evidence, where the "if, then" relationships have been demonstrated to be effective.

Working with an intervention or prevention program that is not based on a proven theory of change is one of the key failings of many programs. The most famous of these failures is the First Lady of the United States, Nancy Reagan's 1982 "Just say no" campaign. The school drug use prevention program known as Drug Abuse Resistance Education (D.A.R.E.) was based on this. With this program, uniformed police officers went into schools to warn students about the dangers of drugs. The officers usually did this once a week during a class time. The program was not based on evidence and it was subsequently found not to be effective and in some cases it may have increased the risk of alcohol and tobacco use (Lilienfeld & Arkowitz, 2014).

According to Johnson et al. (1988), the theories that attempt to explain behavior changes are primarily based in psychology. Previously, the study of substance use prevention was similar to the study of epidemiology and explored antecedents and correlates related to substance use. Johnson et al. (1988) provided one of the early summaries of the theories attempting to explain substance use.

More recently, the European Monitoring Centre for Drugs and Drug Addiction (EMCDDA) produced a handbook for decision makers involved in prevention and within this a summary of theories was provided along with examples (EMCDDA, 2019). According to the EMCDDA (2019, p. 44), it is important to have a basic understanding of the current theories if one is planning on developing an intervention or prevention program. Programs need to be based on what is known as, empirically driven theory, that is, theories that have been proven through data-driven research.

An overview of important prevention theories is provided in Table 4.3, courtesy of the EMCDDA (EMCDDA, 2019).

Once a theory or a selection of theories have been chosen for a program then a logic model of expected outcomes based on the theory can be developed. According to CES (2022), a logic model is a tool usually in the form of a table or a figure that captures a description of the situation and defines agreed inputs, outputs or activities, that is key tasks and areas of work that help achieve the desired and expected outcomes. The logic model should include a description of short-, medium-, and longer-term outcomes. These outcomes are the intended or unintended changes that occur because of the intervention or program.

A publicly available template for a logic model is provided for downloading and sharing by Evaluation Support Scotland (2020) and is adapted here for illustration in Fig. 4.1. The link for the interactive template is provided within the references.

Cultural Adaptation and Fidelity

The UNODC and the World Health Organization (WHO, 2018) provide a comprehensive report on international standards for drug use prevention within which the international scientific evidence is summarized. They emphasize that most of the studies of prevention are conducted in high income countries including North America, Europe, and Oceania. Few studies exist within other cultural settings and prior to the implementation of existing programs into newer diverse setting it is important to consider culture within the situational analysis. While fidelity to the original program is essential, a cultural adaptation may be required.

Fidelity is the delivering of an evidence-based intervention exactly as intended by those who developed it (CES, 2022). Fidelity can be enhanced by ensuring the program or intervention is manualized. That is, a manual of the components of the program and how to deliver them is available either in hard copy or online.

Adaptation of existing programs in new settings is discussed by WHO (2018) who advise, a careful, systematic adaptation of the program within the new setting

Table 4.3 Overview of some important prevention theories

General theories	Year	Description
Bandura's social learning theory	1977	Humans learn behavior by observing others and imitating and modelling these behaviors
Jessor and Jessor's problem behavior theory	1977	Multiple risky behaviors have the same or common root or base and these are influenced by the interaction of the individual with their environment
Bronfenbrenner's ecology of human development	1979	Systems or contexts outside the individual and how they influence individual behavior
Ajzen's theory of planned behavior	1991	There is a link between attitudes and behavior and three sets of perceptions/attitudes guide behavior: Beliefs about the outcomes or consequences of the behavior Beliefs about others' normative expectations (or social acceptability) of the behavior Beliefs about the barriers to and enhancers of the performance of the behavior
Prevention-specific theories	Year	Description
Flay and Petraitis' theory of triadic influence	2003	Three influences contribute to risky behavior: Cultural factors (e.g., the perceived tolerance for adolescent alcohol use) Social or interpersonal factors (e.g., having parents who use substances) Intrapersonal factors (e.g., poor impulse control)
Hawkins and colleagues' risk and protective factors	1992	Risks of substance use are divided into societal and cultural factors that provide the legal and normative expectations of behavior and intra- and inter-personal factors (families, school classrooms, and peers)
Catalano and colleagues' positive youth development	1999	It is important to enhance and reinforce positive development
Werner and Smith's resilience theory	1982	Some individuals have special abilities to adapt to stressful situations and events
Biglan and Hinds' nurturing environments	2009	This combines many aspects of these other theories and focuses on risk reduction and the promotion of resilience and other positive attributes

(Adapted from Table 2, (EMCDDA, 2019) EMCDDA, European Prevention Curriculum, p. 45)

ideally in collaboration with the original program developers. The adapted program should be monitored and evaluated with a control group with a monitoring of pre- and post-outcomes like those outcomes measured in the original program. This will allow for comparability of outcomes in the culturally adapted program.

Fig. 4.1 A logic model template. (Note a publicly available template for use is available at https://evaluationsupportscotland.org.uk/wp-content/uploads/2020/08/final_signed_off_interactive_logic_model_template.pdf)

<table>
<tr><th>Inputs
(These will be intervention or program specific)</th><th>Activities
(These should build upon the inputs)</th><th colspan="3">Outcomes
(These should reflect aspects of the theory or theories underpinning the intervention)</th></tr>
<tr><td></td><td></td><td>Short term outcomes</td><td>Medium term outcomes</td><td>Longer term impacts</td></tr>
<tr><td></td><td></td><td colspan="3">The level (individual, family, setting, community, local or national etc) at which these are measured will depend on the interventions short, medium and longer term aims and objectives.</td></tr>
<tr><td></td><td></td><td></td><td></td><td></td></tr>
<tr><td></td><td></td><td></td><td></td><td></td></tr>
<tr><td></td><td></td><td></td><td></td><td></td></tr>
<tr><td colspan="2">Assumptions</td><td colspan="3">External factors</td></tr>
<tr><td colspan="2"></td><td colspan="3"></td></tr>
</table>

Conclusion and Sample Prevention Registry

Prevention and intervention strategies need to be age appropriate, evidence based and informed by theory. Implementation must consider cultural settings yet fidelity to the original program is essential. The development of an agreed logic model reflecting the underlying theory is required to ensure the monitoring and evaluation of inputs, output, and expected outcomes. A manualized program containing all these program details, will enhance fidelity. Registries of evaluated programs within differing settings, addressing varying age groups, risk factors or substances are available. One example, the Xchange Prevention Registry, provides a ranking of the available evidence for the program and is available at https://www.emcdda.europa.eu/best-practice/xchange_en.

Two case studies illustrating prevention programs are provided below.

Case Study 4.1: Selective Secondary Prevention: A Parenting Intervention for Early Childhood Behavioral Problems

Introduction

McGilloway et al. (2012) highlight that early childhood behavioral problems are predictive of anti-social behavior in youth and criminal behavior, poor employment prospects, and mental ill health in adulthood. Nawi et al. (2021) have also highlighted that poor emotional regulation, behavioral problems, having psychiatric disorders such as conduct problems and negative upbringing with poor parenting skills are risk factors for substance use. At a community level they have found that community poverty is also a risk factor.

Interventions which address these known risk factors which are founded in research evidence and are underpinned by relevant theory are needed to reduce the impact of the risk factors and enhance protectors. An example of one such program is the Incredible Years Basic Parenting Program (IYBP). A series of related programs have also been developed and their details and underlying theories are described by Webster-Stratton (2005). The programs also follow a developmental approach as outlined by UNODC and WHO (WHO, 2018).

One urban disadvantaged community, Archways (https://archways.ie/) supported by philanthropic funding decided to implement an Incredible Years program for its community. The aim of the intervention was to assess the effectiveness of the Incredible Years Basic Parenting Program (Webster-Stratton, 2005) within an urban disadvantage community of parents with children experiencing persistent behavioral problems. The program originally contained 12–18 group-based sessions and was based on behavioral and social learning theories. The current program consisted of 14 sessions, was manualized and was delivered face to face with parents. Childcare and other supports were provided to enable parents to attend the sessions.

Methods

The evaluation of the program was conducted by McGilloway et al. (2012). Parents were included if their child was aged between 32 and 88 months and if the child scored above a clinical cutoff on the Eyberg Child Behavior Inventory (ECBI). Participants (n = 149) were randomly allocated on a 2:1 ratio to an intervention group (n = 103) or a control group (n = 46). For ethical reasons the control group also received the intervention after the randomized control trial was completed.

Child behavior, parenting skills, and parent well-being were measured at baseline and at a 6-month follow-up point. To ensure fidelity to the program, the facilitators of parent groups receiving the intervention received standardized training on the program delivery and the centers where the intervention was delivered were supported by staff with background training in psychology, counselling, education, and related relevant fields. Fidelity to the program was monitored by a weekly facilitator competed checklist. This enabled the facilitators to check that they had covered the relevant material for the week and that parents had completed their related exercises.

Attendance at the group sessions was also monitored to assess treatment dosage. This attendance monitoring enabled the evaluators to assess how much of the program parents received and how this might impact upon desired outcomes.

Results

McGilloway et al. (2012) found statistically significant differences in child disordered behavior with the intervention group showing improvements as measured by the ECBI Intensity and Problem subscales. Similar improvements for the intervention group were found within the child hyperactive-inattentive behaviors and social competence measures. Parent competencies and well-being were also improved for parents within the intervention groups.

Taking baseline readings into account an analysis of covariance found significant intervention—control group differences on the Strengths and Difficulties Questionnaire, total difficulties scores. Significant intervention effects were also found at follow-up on parent-reported levels of hyperactivity and inattention and on prosocial behavior. Analysis of the observations of child positive behaviors did not show significance but observed child problem behavior in the intervention group was significant when compared with the control group.

Findings on fidelity to the program showed that 90% of all materials had been covered within the 14 sessions. Facilitators also reported that parents completed or attempted their exercises and activities for 73% of the 14 sessions. Approximately three quarters (76%) of the first cohort of participants attended seven or more sessions (mean attendance was 10.8 sessions) compared with half (52%) of the second cohort (mean attendance was 6.6 sessions). In total, 31% of participants attended three or fewer sessions. Reasons for non-attendance included illness, work commitments, and concerns about privacy and ethos of the program (Furlong & McGilloway, 2012).

Discussion

Although the Incredible Years Basic Parenting Program was developed within a United States setting the evaluation of the IYBP within one of the first European settings showed that the program was transferable and remained effective. The program was delivered in a European urban disadvantaged setting, facilitated by community-based services in a new cultural environment.

The strengths of program delivery and the evaluation included the fidelity to the program design, the training of the facilitators, the child support for parents and the evidence-based nature, theory informed and developmental approach of the program which targeted known risk and protective factors. These known factors while not explicitly expressed in a logic model were objectively measured pre and post the intervention using internationally, reliable, and comparable scales.

Limitations however included the sustainability of the program delivery given costs of staff, childcare, and training of staff on program delivery. This program was evaluated within a pragmatic, community based, randomized control trial and this too may have had a positive effect on outcomes. Nevertheless, the results as measured in the short-term were positive.

Case Study 4.2: Universal Primary Prevention Using a Whole School Approach in Middle Childhood

Introduction

Within the developmental approach of the UNODC and WHO (WHO, 2018) international standards on drug use prevention, the middle childhood stage is identified. This is the stage after early childhood education which includes children of 2–5 years of age. Middle childhood comes before early adolescence. Within middle childhood children begin to spend more time away from their home and family and increasing time with their peers within a school environment. It is at this time that school culture and education become increasingly important in the child's development. Social skill, prosocial behavior, impulse, and self-control become protective factors.

To enhance protective factors, parenting skills programs, personal and social skills education in school, classroom environment improvement programs, policies to retain children in school and finally addressing mental health disorders are all important interventions at this developmental stage. The school setting is an ideal place to implement universal primary prevention for children within this age group.

The Prevention Action Alliance (2023) summarizing information from the United States Substance Abuse Mental Health Service Administration (SAMHSA) (SAMHSA, 2015) provides a listing of six key strategies for universal/primary prevention. These are:

1. Dissemination of information to provide the population with awareness and knowledge of the nature and extent of drug misuse and its effects.
2. Education where the teacher and participants interact with each other, this improves the life and social skills of participants.
3. Suggesting of alternatives provides activities that don't include drugs, including alcohol and tobacco, in hopes that participants will have their needs met without resorting to drugs.
4. Environmental changes to establish community standards, codes, and attitudes to influence the misuse of drugs in a community.
5. Introducing processes based in the community with a view to enabling a community to provide prevention and treatment services.
6. Establishing problem identification and referral processes, this involves identifying people who have initiated drug misuse to assess if their behavior can be changed through education. As this is a prevention activity it does not refer people to treatment but provides intervention before treatment is needed.

The World Health Organization defines a health promoting school as one in which, "all members of the school community work together to provide pupils with integrated and positive experiences and structures which promote and protect their health" (Lahiff, 2008, pp. citing WHO, 1997). The Childhood Development Initiative (CDI) is a registered charity with a mission "to improve outcomes for children by delivering quality, integrated, evidence-informed services and workforce development through partnership and innovation" (Childhood Development Initiative, 2021). As part of this mission, the CDI developed and implemented a healthy school's program in five middle schools within the disadvantaged region it served.

The Healthy Schools Program of CDI was developed locally and manualized (Lahiff, 2002, 2008). The manual provided the research from which the program was constructed (both the international health promoting schools' literature and local context research) as well as practical guidelines setting out a road map for the schools. The manual presented a logic model that provided a framework for the program and outlined anticipated outcomes and indicators of success from the healthy school initiative.

Methods

The focus of the program was on addressing processes (policy, procedures, and practice) that facilitated change, leading a more health-promoting school environment. The work was completed with the support of a school-based healthy schools coordinator, whose role was to guide the program by supporting schools to develop their capacity to address areas of health in accordance with each school's uniquely identified needs and priorities. To identify these needs and priorities, a support systems checklist was set out in the Healthy Schools manual to assist the coordinator and the school community (staff, families, and children) to classify areas that were working successfully in the school and those that could be developed by the school community and the coordinator.

Working with national, community, family, and school stakeholders, the healthy school's coordinator supported the school to develop sustained processes for the development of health-promoting school environments with the aim of improving child health and well-being outcomes and building future resilience.

A comprehensive evaluation of the program was conducted exploring both the processes of implementation and the impacts in terms of child, family, and school outcomes (Comiskey et al., 2012). The sample in the impact evaluation consisted of children from five intervention schools ($N = 467$) and two comparison schools ($N = 137$).

Short-term health indicators included absenteeism (school records), immunization and dental uptake (official records) rates. Long-term health outcomes included Health Related Quality of Life (HRQoL, Kidscreen-27), depressive symptoms

(Children's Depression Inventory), risky health behaviors (Health Related Behavior Questionnaire, HRBQ), and a computation of body mass index (BMI).

Additional demographic information was obtained from each child using a demographic profile questionnaire. Responses for younger children in Junior and Senior infant classes (aged 4–6 years) were obtained from parents. Results from intervention and comparison schools were compared and tested for differences each year.

Data for the process evaluation included a series of semi- structured interviews with principals and parents, focus groups with teachers, independent observation at school meetings and documentary analysis of governance and administration meetings. Data were analyzed using an inductive, bottom-up thematic analysis approach of Braun and Clarke (2006); Clarke et al. (2015).

Additional data was captured through a selection of child participatory methods with a smaller sample of children and a simple set of children's drawings requested from 220 children aged 8–12 years. These children were asked to draw a picture of their family, and all were given similar pencils and blank paper. A simple visual content analysis was used to analyze the drawings.

Results

Over 600 children in five intervention and two comparison schools were recruited. The impact and process evaluation findings are detailed by Comiskey et al. (2015). The impact evaluation found that while changes were being seen in the schools' approach to improving the health and well-being of children, there were no statistically significant changes in the children's outcomes. The process evaluation sought to understand why no changes were observed in the intervention schools. Through the interviews it was revealed that prior to implementing the program the dedicated manual for the program outlining the necessary steps was not available.

In terms of decision-making, it was found that top-down decision-making based on the surrounding community needs as opposed to bespoke school needs were made. While all schools were within a disadvantaged region one schools needs may have been school absenteeism, another may have been child obesity or school bullying. The "one-size-fits-all" all approach of the program did not meet the individual school needs. This was compounded by the lack of availability of the manual and the completion of the school checklist prior to the program implementation.

The selection of children's participatory method drawings revealed that families varied and while parents may have been considered the target for the implementation of the "whole school approach," parents were not always the person in the child's life who provided the daily health-related support to the child. Often grandparents, aunts or extended family may have had a central role in daily activities (Hollywood et al., 2021).

The wider sample of children's drawings revealed large families with varying family members and pets in a range of family settings (Shimer et al., 2014). An example of one of the children's drawings can be found in Fig. 4.2.

Discussion

The findings from the evaluation of this healthy schools' universal primary intervention program were disappointing given the program was manualized, theory-based with an appropriate logic model.

Given that adopting the principles of a "healthy school" takes time and that most health indicators should be measured over the long term, the literature suggests that expectations of outcome changes in the short-term should remain low (Comiskey et al., 2012). However, the key failing of this program was not necessarily the program itself, but rather its implementation. Sufficient time was not provided for the

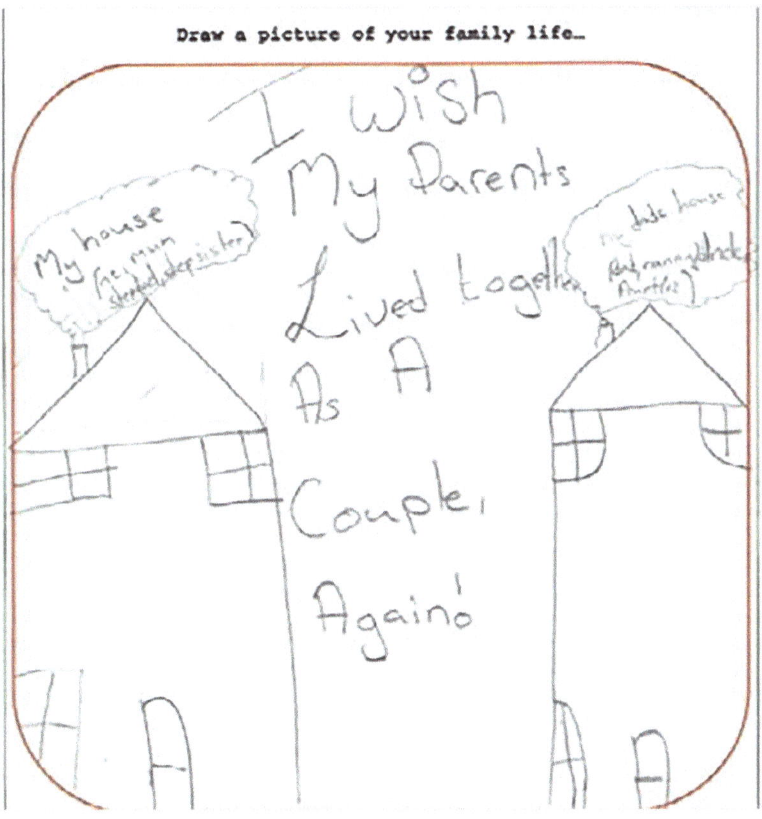

Fig. 4.2 A child's drawings illustrating their family life

manual to be ready; teachers were not trained on the program implementation and this task was left to a sole healthy schools' coordinator. Staff within schools are key drivers of school policy and programs, and increasing their capacity through training is essential for successful implementation (Rowling, 2009).

The schools did not target their specific needs and checklists identifying these were not ready when the program was started and were subsequently not completed. The successful implementation required sufficient lead-in time to ensure that each school was ready in terms of its understanding. Furthermore, healthy schools' coordinators roles needed to be clarified as facilitators of development and change rather than as unsustainable providers of health activities.

This case study provides a good example of how an established program which worked in other settings will not necessarily work in another if sufficient preparatory work is not provided in advance of implementation (Lee et al., 2006). Further details on the stages, enablers, and barriers to implementing a range of programs or polices are provided in Chap. 10.

References

Braun, V., & Clarke, V. (2006). Using thematic analysis in psychology. *Qualitative Research in Psychology, 3*(2), 77–101. https://doi.org/10.1191/1478088706qp063oa

CAST. (2023). *Insight North East Asia.* Retrieved November 20, 2023, from Insight_NEA_Apr25_V3.pdf (asiapacific.ca)

CES. (2022). *An introductory guide to implementation.* Retrieved December 13, 2023, from https://implementation.effectiveservices.org/

Childhood Development Initiative. (2021). *CDI vision and mission 2021.* Retrieved November 14, 2023, from https://www.cdi.ie/about-us/mission-statement

Clarke, V., Braun, V., & Hayfield, N. (2015). Thematic analysis. In J. A. Smith (Ed.), *Qualitative psychology: A practical guide to research methods* (3rd ed.). Sage.

Comiskey, C. M., O'Sullivan, K., Quirke, M. B., Wynne, C., Kelly, P., & McGilloway, S. (2012). *Evaluation of the effectiveness of the childhood development initiative's healthy schools programme* (ISBN: 978-0-9570232-4-6). https://www.cdi.ie/wp-content/uploads/2016/11/CDI-HSP-Report-12.11-web.pdf.

Comiskey, C. M. O'Sullivan, K., Quirke, M., Wynne, C., Hollywood, E and McGilloway, S. (2015). *An analysis of the first implementation and impact of the World Health Organisation Health Promoting School Model within urban disadvantaged schools in Ireland.* Vulnerable Children and Youth Studies DOI:10.1080/17450128.2015.1080394 Available at https://www.tandfonline.com/doi/epdf/10.1080/17450128.2015.1080394 accessed 14th November, 2023.

EMCDDA. (2019). *European Prevention Curriculum (EUPC): A handbook for decision-makers, opinion-makers and policy-makers in science-based pre-vention of substance use.* Retrieved November 13, 2023, from https://www.emcdda.europa.eu/publications/manuals/european-prevention-curriculum_en

EMCDDA and Europol. (2023). *EU drug markets: In-depth analysis.* Retrieved August 28, 2023 from https://www.emcdda.europa.eu/publications/eu-drug-markets_en

Evaluation Support Scotland. (2020). *ESS evaluation tool: Interactive logic model template.* Retrieved November 13, 2023, from https://evaluationsupportscotland.org.uk/wp-content/uploads/2020/08/final_signed_off_interactive_logic_model_template.pdf

Furlong, M., & McGilloway, S. (2012). The incredible years parenting program in Ireland: A qualitative analysis of the experience of disadvantaged parents. *Clinical Child Psychology and Psychiatry, 17*(4), 616–630.

Hollywood, E., Comiskey, C., Lalor, J., & Creaner, M. (2021, March 10–11). *What does family mean for the school-aged child who lives in an area of urban disadvantage?* Trinity health and education inter-national research conference (THEconf2021), online.

Johnson, E. M., Amatetti, S., Funkhouser, J. E., & Johnson, S. (1988). Theories and models supporting prevention approaches to alcohol problems among youth. *Public Health Reports, 103*(6), 578.

Kisling, L. A., & Das, M. J. (2023, January). *Prevention strategies. [updated 2023 Aug 1].* StatPearls [internet]. Treasure Island (FL): StatPearls Publishing. https://www.ncbi.nlm.nih.gov/books/NBK537222/

Lahiff, J. (2002). The development of a health-promoting school model in Ireland. In B. B. Jensen & V. Simovska (Eds.), *Models of health-promoting schools in Europe*. WHO Regional Office for Europe.

Lahiff, J. (2008). TWCDI healthy schools manual.

Lee, A., Cheng, F., Fung, Y., et al. (2006). Can Health Promoting Schools contribute to the better health and wellbeing of young people? The Hong Kong experience. *Journal of Epidemiology Community Health, 60*, 530–536.

Lilienfeld, S. O., & Arkowitz, H. (2014). *Why "just say no" Doesn't work.* Scientific American. Retrieved November 13, 2023, from https://www.scientificamerican.com/article/why-just-say-no-doesnt-work/

Malick, R. (2018). Prevention of substance use disorders in the community and workplace. *Indian Journal of Psychiatry, 60*(Suppl 4), S559. Retrieved November 11, 2023, from https://nida.nih.gov/publications/drugs-brains-behavior-science-addiction/drug-misuse-addiction

Martins, C., Godycki-Cwirko, M., Heleno, B., & Brodersen, J. (2018). Quaternary prevention: Reviewing the concept: Quaternary prevention aims to protect patients from medical harm. *European Journal of General Practice, 24*(1), 106–111.

McGilloway, S., et al. (2012). A parenting intervention for childhood behavioral problems: A randomized controlled trial in disadvantaged community-based settings. *Journal of Consulting and Clinical Psychology, 80*(1), 116–127. https://doi.org/10.1037/a0026304

Nawi, A. M., Ismail, R., Ibrahim, F., Hassan, M. R., Manaf, M. R. A., Amit, N., Ibrahim, N., & Shafurdin, N. S. (2021). Risk and protective factors of drug abuse among adolescents: A systematic review. *BMC Public Health, 21*, 1–15.

NIDA. (2012). *Principles of drug addiction treatment: A research-based guide.* Retrieved November 20, 2023, from https://www.drugabuse.gov/sites/default/files/podat_1.pdf

NIDA. (2021). *Drug overdose deaths in 2020 were horrifying*. National Institute on Drug Abuse, Advancing Addiction Science. Retrieved January 19, 2024 from https://www.scientificamerican.com/article/drug-overdose-deaths-in-2020-were-horrifying/

Paradigma Youth Coalition. (2023). *Youth response to the 2023 world drug report.* Retrieved November 10, 2023, from https://www.drugsandalcohol.ie/39442/1/Youth-Response-2023-World-Drug-Report%20%281%29.pdf

Pattojoshi, A., & Tikka, S. K. (2020). School-based substance use disorder prevention in India: A brief appraisal. *Indian Journal of Psychiatry, 62*(4), 427. Retrieved November 10, 2023, from https://doi.org/10.4103/psychiatry.IndianJPsychiatry_43_19.

Prevention Action Alliance. (2023). *Learn About Prevention.* Retrieved November 10, 2023, from https://preventionactionalliance.org/resources/about-prevention/

Rowling, L. (2009). Strengthening "school" in school mental health promotion. *Health Education, 109*(4), 357–368.

SAMHSA. (2015). *Adults with attention deficit hyperactivity dis-order and substance use disorders*. Substance Abuse and Mental Health Services Administration. Retrieved September 1, 2023 from https://store.samhsa.gov/sites/default/files/d7/priv/sma15-4925.pdf

Shimer, J., Comiskey, C. M., Tobin, C., & Banka, P. (2014). *The healthy schools Programme: Taking a deeper look into the lives of disadvantaged children through visual content analysis.* Research report for the University of New Hampshire Summer Internship and Inquiry Journal. Retrieved December 14, 2023, from https://scholars.unh.edu/inquiry_2015/4/

UNODC. (2023a). *United nations office on drugs and crime (2023) world drug report*. Retrieved August 2, 2023 from https://www.unodc.org/unodc/en/press/releases/2023a/June/unodc-world-drug-report-2023-warns-of-converging-crises-as-illicit-drug-markets-continue-to-expand.html?testme

UNODC. (2023b). *United nations office on drugs and crime: World drug report 2023*. United Nations. Retrieved August 2, 2023 from https://www.unodc.org/unodc/en/press/releases/2023b/June/unodc-world-drug-report-2023-warns-of-converging-crises-as-illicit-drug-markets-continue-to-expand.html?testme

Webster-Stratton, C. (2005). The incredible years: A training series for the prevention and treatment of conduct problems in young children. In E. D. Hibbs & P. S. Jensen (Eds.), *Psychosocial treatments for child and adolescent disorders: Empirically based strategies for clinical practice* (2nd ed., pp. 507–555). American Psychological Association.

WHO. (1997). *Promoting Health through Schools*. Report of a WHO Expert Committee on Comprehensive School Health Education and Promotion. WHO Technical Report Series 870, Geneva: World Health Organization.

WHO. (2018). *International standards on drug use prevention* (2nd ed.). Retrieved November 13, 2023, from https://www.unodc.org/documents/prevention/UNODC-WHO_2018_prevention_standards_E.pdf

Chapter 5
Outreach, Treatment, and Recovery: Understanding and Evaluating an Outreach, Treatment or Recovery Intervention

Setting the Scene

> *I began using substances from quite a young age—by the age of 16 I was smoking crack cocaine and then by 17 I was fully dependent on heroin. I got into problems and had to leave my hometown and found myself homeless. I ended up in temporary accommodation and went through the whole hostel system. Eventually I managed to get my own place and linked in with the support services I needed.*
>
> *Now I volunteer in the Needle Exchange and Street Injectors Support Service in Belfast three to four times a week. We go out around the streets doing outreach work—sometimes we would find people in car parks that could be dying due to overdose. We use a drug called Naloxone to reverse overdose and administer first aid as well...... Winning the Northern Ireland Volunteer of the Year Award was mind-blowing.*

Neil Potter, Volunteer, Drug Outreach Team, eXtern, Belfast Northern Ireland. Reproduced from https://www.extern.org/neils-story-drug-outreach-team

Introduction

Treatment works. As with all health issues, when treatment is based on scientific evidence and addresses patient needs, improvements are expected. Similarly, it has been established through a range of international studies that evidence-based substance use treatment that addresses the needs of clients is effective in reducing substance use and improving lives (C. M. Comiskey et al., 2023). In addition to reducing substance use, treatment also saves money (WHO and UNODC, 2020). According to NIDA (2012) the rate of savings to investment can be over 12:1, with every one dollar spent on substance use treatment, over 12 dollars can be saved. Savings occur through reductions in healthcare usage, reductions in drug-related crime, and savings in the costs of criminal justice systems.

C. Comiskey, *Addiction Research and Evaluation*, Advances in Mental Health and Addiction, https://doi.org/10.1007/978-3-031-65917-1_5

As with other health conditions, substance use, and substance use disorders can be described on a continuum from low to high severity with varying levels of complexity. These levels can be further complicated by additional demographic, social, physical, and mental health factors. For example, the treatment needs of a postpartum mother using excessive alcohol and caring for her newborn baby can be very different to the needs of a homeless man who is displaced, seeking international protection, dealing with trauma and possibly using opioids.

Similarly, clients who have been in treatment and are in long-term recovery may be at a more advanced stage of their treatment and recovery journey. While this journey as experienced by an individual may not be linear and people may move between stages, there is an internationally recognized hierarchy in the provision of services given the stage the patient/client is currently within.

A diversity of treatment approaches is needed, and these are described within this chapter. This chapter also provides guidance on how to evaluate treatment; how to decide what is important to measure; where to access data for your evaluation and how many clients you may need in your evaluation. Finally, two case studies are provided as examples.

Levels of Treatment and Recovery Services

Rush (2010) provides a historical and developmental overview of treatment approaches. This varies from the continuum of care model, which was an advancement on the "one-size-fits-all" approach, to a system of care that embraces a more holistic tiered approach. The continuum of care model was structured with categories of specialized services ideally with clients passing through these various treatments and settings.

For example, a client may move through intake, screening, withdrawal management/detoxification, stabilization, assessment and treatment planning, treatment intervention of varying intensity and finally continuing care. This continuum was further developed to include recovery monitoring and checkup. The idea of a stepped care model was based on this continuum, whereby a client could, once they were assessed, be assigned to the least intensive step of this model. Clients could then step up to a more intensive care treatment if outcomes were not improved or step down to a less intensive treatment if outcomes were positive.

While the continuum of care model remains useful its key limitation is its lack of linkage of the treatment services to wider health, social, justice, and education supports and services. Yet these are the very services that are required within an integrated substance use treatment system if it is to meet the needs of its diversity of clients (Babor et al., 2010).

A system of care framework with a tiered approach was adopted by the English, National Treatment Agency for Substance Use (National Treatment Agency, 2002). This model defined a set of tiers aligned with problem severity, its aim was to locate various aspects of the comprehensive treatment system within the tiers and then work with local areas over time to address system gaps through funding and more integrated policies and care planning (National Treatment Agency, 2002).

A revised model was developed for clarity in 2006 (National Treatment Agency for Substance Misuse, 2006) and this defined the four tiers of the model on the basis of interventions to be offered within them, what these interventions were, the settings in which they may be found, and the competencies required by staff in the services for these interventions to be offered to clients and their families. A summary of this four-tiered model is provided in Table 5.1.

A tiered system of care for substance use has been widely adopted and further examples and developments with needs-based planning can be seen within the Canadian healthcare system (Rush et al., 2019; Rush et al., 2014).

Table 5.1 A summary of the National Treatment Agencies (2006) tiered treatment system

	Summary of tiered treatment system
Tier 1	Interventions include provision of drug-related information and advice, screening, and referral to specialized drug treatment Tier 1 interventions are provided in the context of general healthcare settings (liver units, antenatal wards, accident and emergency and pharmacies), or social care, education or criminal justice settings (probation, courts, prison reception) where the focus is not drug treatment
Tier 2	Interventions include provision of drug-related information and advice, triage assessment, referral to structured drug treatment, brief psychosocial interventions, harm reduction interventions (including needle exchange) and aftercare Tier 2 interventions may be delivered separately from Tier 3 but will often also be delivered in the same setting and by the same staff as Tier 3 interventions. Other settings to increase access are through outreach, pharmacy settings and criminal justice settings
Tier 3	Interventions include provision of community-based specialized drug assessment and coordinated care planned treatment and drug specialist liaison Tier 3 interventions are normally delivered in specialized drug treatment services with their own premises in the community or on hospital sites. Other delivery may be by outreach. Tier 3 interventions may be delivered alongside Tier 2 interventions Some may be based in primary care settings (shared care schemes and GP-led prescribing services), as well as pharmacies, but drug specialist-led services are required within the local systems for the provision of care for severe or complex needs and to support primary care Drug treatment interventions for offenders may be delivered in prison settings and community criminal justice programs are delivered in contracted community drug treatment services (statutory or voluntary) or in-house by probation staff on probation premises
Tier 4	Interventions include provision of residential specialized drug treatment, which is care planned and care coordinated to ensure continuity of care and aftercare Ideal settings to provide inpatient drug detoxification and stabilization are specialized dedicated inpatient or residential substance misuse units or wards Continuity of care is essential for preserving gains achieved in residential treatments. Therefore, there is an argument for providing inpatient detoxification beds attached to residential rehabilitation units provided there are adequate medical supports Within prisons, specialist detoxification units, therapeutic communities (drug specific) and some (residential) 12-step programs are Tier 4 interventions

Barker et al. (2016) developed the model within the Australian system and instead of using the concepts of substance use severity through acuity, chronicity, and complexity they measured problem severity using objective measurements. They used the Alcohol Use Disorder Identification Test and Drug Use Disorder Identification Test scores) and complexity scores (as indicated by high psychological distress, housing instability, and an absence of meaningful activity) (Barker et al., 2016).

The American Society for Addiction Medicine (ASAM) also recognize that treatment isn't a one-size-fits-all solution and that each client has unique needs which can include co-occurring mental illness, psychological problems, social problems with family and community or housing and vocational challenges with work, legal or educational difficulties.

The American Society for Addiction Medicine has identified five tiers of care starting with the first tier which is known as level 0.5 up to the fifth tier known as level 4. Various sublevels within these exist and the aim of these levels is to help people find the best care to meet their needs. People can move between levels and can be referred to higher or lower levels as needed. These tiers are described in Table 5.2.

The international standards for the treatment of drug use disorders (WHO and UNODC, 2020) also stresses that drug treatment services need to meet the needs of the target group and a range of different treatment approaches are required. They too stress that no single type of treatment is suitable for all types, severities or stages of drug use and drug use disorders. Services not only need to provide for drug use disorders, but services are also needed which address within communities

Table 5.2 The five levels of the tiered system of care as outlined by ASAM (Mosel, 2023)

Tiered system of care (ASAM)
0.5 Prevention/Early intervention
1 Outpatient services
2 Intensive outpatient/Partial hospitalization
Intensive outpatient services
Partial hospitalization services
3 Residential/Inpatient services
Clinically managed low-intensity residential services
Clinically managed population-specific high-intensity residential services
Clinically managed high-intensity residential services
Medically monitored high-intensity inpatient services
4 Medically managed intensive inpatient services

interventions aimed at reducing the negative health, social and justice consequences of substance use. A range of treatments or interventions need to be in place in varying settings and these include outreach, outpatient, inpatient, and residential care settings. Outreach services are discussed initially.

Outreach Services

As it may be many years between when a person first uses a substance and when they may need or seek treatment, outreach services are an essential part of a national or regional treatment system. The role of outreach is to proactively seek contact with people who use substances to motivate them to engage with services, reduce harm or to minimize negative health and social effects of substance use. People working in outreach services establish initially informal contacts and can aim to reach other people effected by the persons substance use, these may be sexual partners or needle sharing contacts. The approach aims to make people who use substances become more motivated to use healthcare and social services, including treatment for substance use disorders. This is the result of new, positive experiences between the individual and the outreach worker and this positive experience that may be in contrast to former experiences which may have been stigmatizing and without a health-led, human rights-based approach (WHO and UNODC, 2020).

Outreach services are designed to serve people who may be considered hard to reach or who may be hidden due to stigma, fear, cultural norms, or other reasons. This may include mothers who use substances but are also experiencing domestic abuse, people seeking international protection, homeless people, people with co-occurring mental health challenges, people who are engaged in sex work, isolated farmers, rural or industrial workers or young urban dwellers. The goal of outreach according to WHO and UNODC (WHO and UNODC, 2020) is to identify target populations, engage them and provide them with unconditional community-based services and interventions including harm reduction interventions.

Rush and Furlong (2020) provide a review of what they term rapid access models for substance use services which includes outreach and WHO and UNODC (2020) provide summaries of the varying types of outreach. A collated summary from these is provided in Table 5.3.

The choice of outreach service developed will depend on the needs of the individuals and an effective outreach program should be flexible, adaptive, and sensitive to these needs. This may depend upon patterns of substance use, age, gender, and social situation. It should also guarantee the confidentiality of people involved in its activities. Examples of mobile and assertive outreach are provided within the case studies within this chapter.

Table 5.3 A description of varying outreach approaches

Detached outreach	Detached outreach is work undertaken outside of any agency, such as work on the streets, in bars, clubs, squats or railway stations. This work is mostly mobile and may be done on foot or using a designated vehicle
Peripatetic outreach	Peripatetic outreach is work undertaken in settings: where people are either already accessing some services (such as needle and syringe programs), or where it is highly likely to encounter target populations (for example prisons, brothels, shelters for homeless people or housing projects) Instead of focusing on individuals, peripatetic outreach focuses on organizations and settings where target populations can be found
Domiciliary outreach	Domiciliary outreach is work undertaken in the homes of target populations. This is important in areas where there are no street drug scenes, or where people who use drugs are isolated from their communities because of stigma and discrimination. Domiciliary outreach involves regular visits to the homes of people who use substances
Assertive outreach	Outreach efforts can fall on a continuum from opportunistic to more assertive, with assertive community treatment (ACT) representing the most formalized, structured and proactive model of outreach. The proactive approach is the key feature of assertive outreach

Evaluating Treatment and Recovery, Assessing Impact

It is recognized that treatment works and the research is available to show that evidence-based treatments that meet the needs of clients produce positive impacts and save money (WHO and UNODC, 2020). Large-scale treatment outcome studies have been conducted internationally for many years. Within the United States of America, Simpson (2003) reported on the Drug Abuse Treatment Outcome Study (DATOS). Within Australia, the Australian Treatment Outcome Study was the first large-scale Australian prospective treatment outcome study on people who use heroin (Darke et al., 2005). This study was ongoing 20 years later.

Within England and Wales, Gossop et al. (2000) provided an overview of 5 years of treatment outcome research and stressed the ongoing importance of using evidence to decide how best to allocate resources. In Scotland, the Drug Outcome Research in Scotland (DORIS) study followed a cohort of 1007 opiate users over a period of 33 months (McKeganey et al., 2006). The Research Outcome Study in Ireland Evaluating Drug Treatment Effectiveness (the ROSIE Study) also followed a national cohort of people in treatment for opiate use (Cox & Comiskey, 2007). Within this study it was observed that treatment works, it reduced substance use, improved physical well-being, improved social functioning, and reduced crime (Comiskey et al., 2009). However, this study also noted that longer-term mental health needs were not being addressed. This is perhaps a good example of the importance of continuing to focus on client needs while they continue to engage with treatment.

Key Questions to Consider in Evaluation

The studies above were all large-scale national studies that evaluated a range of different treatment modalities (opiate agonist treatment, needle exchange, detoxification, abstinence-based treatments) different treatment settings (in-patient, out-patient, community, long-term residential) and different regions (urban, rural, city). Not every country, region, locality, or service can conduct such studies given the time and resources needed. We can however learn from these studies, and they provide us with a range of questions we need to consider and decide on when we wish to evaluate our intervention, outreach, treatment, or recovery service. A selection of these is provided in Table 5.4.

How Many Participants Are Needed in an Evaluation to Measure Change?

When planning an evaluation or research study, one of the most common challenges is determining what the sample size should be. While this may seem like a simple question it does not have a quick and easy answer, it is a bit a like asking "how long is a piece of string?" Fortunately, there are some simple steps to follow and some excellent published papers one can use to help answer this question.

Some key decisions must be made before we answer the main question on numbers of participants required, these questions have been addressed in detail in Table 5.4. They are:

- What is the overall study aim and the key objectives? This needs to be stated as clearly as possible. For example, instead of asking, "Does our needle exchange intervention work? "We can ask, "Does our needle exchange intervention reduce daily needle sharing?" Similarly, instead of asking, "Does our school prevention program reduce substance use?" We can ask, "Does our school prevention program increase weekly sports participation time?"
- What are the most important measures or critical variables in the study? From the examples above we have already identified what we believe are the most critical variables.
- What is our level of resources in terms of finances, time, staffing etc. While in theory we may wish to include more participants in our study we may not have the resources available in terms of staffing and time to measure and monitor all the participants.

In comparative studies, that is any study comparing two or more groups the aim is to compare the groups and determine if a difference between them exists, which is not explained by simply choosing samples which were very different. In another example we might wish to compare a person's mental health before and after a treatment, we might have a pre- and post-cohort study design and our key aim is to

Table 5.4 The 12-stepped questions template for evaluation: Important considerations when evaluating an intervention, outreach, treatment or recovery service

Questions	Considerations	Your response
1. What are the primary needs of the people who use our service?	As we saw, the needs of people who use your intervention must come first. While the individual needs of your client group may vary, is there an overarching need that the intervention can address of the client group? For example, in a country where only detoxification is available, is harm reduction a realistic need that should be addressed?	
2. What is the key goal of our service?	Aim to articulate the single primary goal your intervention is aiming to address. For example, if you are providing an intervention to mothers who use substances, is your goal to reduce substance use or is it to enable mothers to keep the care of their children? Ultimately within your intervention you may impact upon both outcomes but is one outcome a primary outcome?	
3. What is the theory or logic model underlying our service and practice provision?	The importance of logic models was discussed within prevention and interventions. Clarifying your logic model and your model of practice or service delivery will help with identifying key outcomes that are expected to change	
4. What domains of outcomes will we measure?	As we have seen earlier in this chapter many domains of a person's life, their family, community, and society can be affected by substance use. These domains include drug use, risk, physical and mental health, quality of life, social functioning, justice, education, and employment. The domains chosen should reflect the logic model	
5. At what level will you measure your key impacts and outcomes within these domains?	Outcomes can be measured at the individual, family, community, and societal levels. For example, within the health domain a key outcome for a needle exchange outreach harm reduction service might be reducing the risk of overdose for their clients. A key outcome for the family might be a reduction in the risk of transmission of HIV or Hepatitis C. A key outcome at the societal level could be a reduction in the usage of acute hospital emergency room services	
6. Is data available to you that measures or captures this data on a regular basis?	Given resources are always under pressure it is good to consider if your key outcomes are already being captured within your service or a related one. For example, if you are providing a schools-based intervention for young people who are currently known to be using substances, is attendance at school one of your key outcomes you wish to improve? If so, then this data is likely to be available. If students and their parents have consented to be involved and have given permission, is there data available in the school nurse records that might provide some pre-intervention or baseline data? Similarly, is there any national registry data or hospital data you can access and select clients from your locality or service?	

(continued)

Table 5.4 (continued)

Questions	Considerations	Your response
7. What tools and instruments will you use to capture the data if it is not readily available?	Do readymade validated and reliable tools, survey instruments already exit that you can use to capture your key outcomes? There are many freely available treatment outcome survey tools or schools-based tools that have been used and tested in a range of settings and countries. Given the level of expertise required to develop a survey it is unwise to attempt this without adequate resources and experience on the team	
8. What are the appropriate and feasible time intervals to capture this data?	The appropriate timing of data capture is essential and should reflect the logic model. If you are measuring change then a pre-intervention or baseline measurement is essential. Within this baseline both historical (over a lifetime, "have you ever," type questions) and recent past (in the last week/month/3 months/6 months/year) type questions will need to be asked. The duration chosen should be carefully selected to be feasible for recall. For example, you might ask "how many overdoses have you experienced within the last 3 months?" It could be difficult to recall beyond that time frame. However, you might ask, "have you attended a hospital emergency department in the last year?" With children you might ask, "what sports have you played in the last week?" Similarly, after baseline and when following up you must consider what is an appropriate duration to follow-up? Is it immediately after the delivery of an intervention? Do you wish to measure immediate change or is immediate change unrealistic? Do you wish to measure short-term and longer-term sustainable changes? If so then 3-, 6-, 12-, or 24-month follow-up periods may be more suitable if resources allow or if an existing longitudinal data registry is available	
9. How will this data be captured?	Will you gather your data online or face to face with interviews or focus groups or will you use observational techniques? Will your data capture be paper-based or will you use a combination of technologies? Do you need specialized equipment to capture the key outcome data? For example, if you are measuring blood pressure do you have trained staff and resources to do this? Have you considered novel ways to capture key data such as visual content analysis, children's drawings or simply "hanging out" as used by many anthropologists?	

(continued)

Table 5.4 (continued)

Questions	Considerations	Your response
10. Where will this data be captured?	Given the nature of the intervention provided where would be suitable locations to capture the data? For example, if you are working with rural women who use substances and experience domestic abuse where will you capture the data? Their homes and localities may not be private, yet they may not have the time or financial resources to travel to meet you. Can you meet them virtually on their phones or are their phones checked and monitored? Can you use a service or a location where the women may already be attending for other reasons? For example, their local public health center or pharmacy? These are challenging questions. If you are working with homeless people, can you meet them in a café and provide them with a meal or is such a location insufficiently private? If you are working with school children, how can you access them without disturbing the school routine and will they participate if they feel their answers may be overheard? If it is feasible, it is considered good practice to allow participants themselves to choose what location suits them best	
11. What is a feasible definition of a participant?	Ideally the definition of a participant in your evaluation should reflect the key impacts and outcomes of your logic model and the target populations of your service. Remembering that target populations do not always refer to people. They can refer to groups of workplaces or industries (you may be providing an intervention on cocaine use to financial institutions or an anti-stigma training program to a group of ministerial departments). To capture appropriate baseline data, you may be restricted in your definition of a participant, you may need to choose only clients who are having their first visit or engagement with your service. However perhaps your service has been in operation a long time and doesn't receive many first-time visitors. In this situation you may need to define a participant as someone who hasn't used your service within the last year. Similarly, within a school setting some students may be attending other interventions within or outside of school that may affect their outcomes within your intervention	
12. How many participants do I need to include in my evaluation to measure effectiveness?	Once the initial answers to the above questions have been addressed as best they can be, you arrive at one of the most challenging questions. The good news is however that once we have answers to the questions above, we can access additional tools to help us answer this all-important question **This final question is addressed in detail in the section below**	

compare the difference in the mean mental health readings of the participants from the two time points. We could use a matched paired *t*-test to do this. If we wished to compare current waiting times for an appointment across three community treatment centers, we might conduct a study with a cross-sectional study design and compare the mean waiting times across the three centers. We could use an analysis of variance (ANOVA) to do this.

Simple explanations and further details on these types of statistics are beyond the scope of this chapter but they are available in summary within Comiskey and Dempsey (2013).

A study may have an overarching aim but perhaps three or four important objectives. We can repeat the sample size estimation for a critical variable for each of the three or four objectives. In practice many variables can be examined in a study and a decision must be made about which variables the calculation is based on and ultimately which estimate will finally be chosen. To choose a variable one solution might be to pick the "most important" variable and to base the calculations for sample size requirements on this.

However, a more realistic approach would be to choose several important variables, perform a separate sample size calculation for each, and then to accept the largest resulting sample size if resources allow for that. If resources do not allow for the largest to be chosen, then a pragmatic approach must be taken and the limitations of this accepted.

The final chosen sample size should also be adjusted to account for non-response rates that is people who may choose not to participate for one reason or another. To ensure we still have an adequate sample size, we can inflate the estimate of the required sample size by 10–20%.

Cohen (1992) has produced a set of tables which provide a guide to the necessary sample sizes for the most frequently used statistical tests. Based on Cohen (1992) a summary table of some key sample sizes calculations are provided in Table 5.5. These have four main assumptions: (1) the data are from a random sample, (2) we test our hypothesis (research question) at the 5% level of significance, (3) we assume a power of 80%, and finally (4) we expect a medium effect. Finally, in practice, resources and finances have a major influence on the sample size chosen. While it may not be possible to achieve the numbers needed for a study, sample size calculations can still provide relevant information about the consequences of the sample size chosen.

In the following section we illustrate through two practical local examples how an intervention can be evaluated.

Further practical details on evaluation design, sample size calculations (power analysis), choosing validated and reliable instruments, retrospective registries, and appropriate data analysis are available (Comiskey et al., 2009, 2012; Comiskey & Snel, 2016).

Table 5.5 A selection of required sample sizes (number of participants needed) given common research and evaluation study designs and assumptions

Study design	Example	Additional assumptions	Sample size	Total sample planned for, given a potential loss of 20%
Comparing the mean reading between two groups	Comparing the mean number of needles used in a week between those attending a needle exchange service and those not attending	The two groups are independent of one another	64 participants in each group	64 + 64 = 128 Add 20% 128 × 1.2 = 154 Plan resources for 160, 80 in each group
Testing for a correlation between two variables	Asking if there is a correlation between the number of times a person attends counselling and their mental health score	There is a linear relationship between the two variables	85 participants in total	85 × 1.2 = 102 Plan resources for a total sample size of 105
Testing for an association (independence) between a binary outcome and a binary attribute	Asking if treatment completion (completed, yes or no) is dependent on having had a prior treatment episode elsewhere (yes or no)		87 participants in total	87 × 1.2 = 105 Plan resources for a total sample size of 110
Comparing the mean reading between three groups	Comparing the mean stress levels between people who attend your service and who are not parents, with those who are parents and live with their children and with those who are parents and do not live with their children		52 participants in each group	52 × 1.2 = 63 63 + 63 + 63 = 189 Plan resources for 198 participants, 66 in each group

Case Study 5.1: Evaluating a Gay Men's Health Outreach Service with a View to Informing the Efficacy, Potential Scale Up, and Roll Out of the Service

Introduction

The findings from the pan-European Internet survey among men who have sex with men (MSM) provided a rationale for online and in-person outreach interventions to address condom access issues, chemsex and levels of STI and HIV testing among survey participants (EMIS, 2019). The Irish National Sexual Health Strategy

2015–2020 also clearly identified gay, bisexual, and MSM as being at increased risk of poorer sexual health outcomes and of contracting STIs and HIV (Healthy Ireland, 2015, p. 31).

The strategy highlighted the epidemiological data related to new HIV cases in Ireland and noted the increase in HIV cases, many of which were occurring amongst MSM and over 50% of which had a delayed or a late diagnosis (Healthy Ireland, 2015, p. 30). The strategy listed interventions such as targeted outreach and condom distribution as potential interventions (Healthy Ireland, 2015, p. 35). Targeted education and outreach is listed as a key recommendation for at risk groups in order to provide positive prevention to mitigate against potential negative sexual health outcomes (Healthy Ireland, 2015, p. 39). A pilot outreach program to address these findings was developed by the Gay Men's Health Service (GMHS) in partnership with the Gay Health Network (GHN).

The objectives of the GMHS outreach program were to:

1. Promote the use of condoms and lube as an effective form of protection from the spread of STIs and HIV and make condoms and lube available.
2. Increase knowledge and awareness about the signs and symptoms of STIs and HIV.
3. Increase awareness about and encourage use of local resources (STI and HIV testing services, information points etc.) for STI and HIV prevention, screening, testing and treatment.
4. Explore and discuss sexual risk assessment and risk reduction, including HIV prevention technologies (PEP, PrEP, undetectable viral load) and STI and HIV testing.
5. Refer to the Man2Man.ie website https://man2man.ie/ for information and/or location-based resources and services that are regionally specific and promote Man2Man.ie and other affiliated related campaigns and materials.
6. Reduce HIV-related stigma.
7. Encourage and support sexual consent and sexual respect, particularly in encounters initiated online.
8. Connect with subpopulations, migrant populations, especially Latin American MSM, and sex workers.

The aim of the evaluation of the pilot program was to provide an evaluation that incorporated the overarching values, philosophy, and context of the four strands of the code of governance which were sex positivity, client-centered service, harm reduction, and skill building and capacity.

The specific objectives were to:

- Assess the ways that the objectives of the program were being achieved.
- Assess the ways in which the outreach program was received by the target audience and other key stakeholders.
- Assess the experience of the outreach service in delivering the program.
- Identify critical success factors and key barriers in relation to implementation.
- Make recommendations for improvements to current operational processes with a focus on resources and reporting data.

Methods

To address these objectives five methodological approaches were taken that included both existing data sources and novel new sources. In summary a multi-method design was chosen which included several quantitative and qualitative approaches to data collection. These five are summarized below:

1. Quantitative analysis of service delivery data (online outreach and in-house clinic data).
2. Quantitative analysis of an on-site survey.
3. Quantitative and qualitative analysis of non-participant structured observation on-site.
4. Qualitative documentary analysis of existing documentary evidence within the service.
5. Qualitative analysis of semi-structured interviews with relevant stakeholders.

Results

The evaluation findings demonstrated that the outreach program was meeting its objectives and operated in line with its stated code of governance. The evaluation found that the main topics addressed in the online outreach sessions were HIV, sexual behavior and sexuality, STIs other than HIV, treatment and mental health, substance use and general information. The overarching topics that were most frequently discussed were STIs other than HIV and related treatment/counselling, followed by HIV and general information.

Within topics discussed, HIV pre-exposure prophylaxis (PrEP) and post-exposure prophylaxis (PEP) were the most frequent individual subjects advised on. It was also found that the service was very efficient and provided on average 20 online individual interactions per week, or approximately one per hour. Extracts from the observation of the live online service (Table 5.6) illustrate some of the findings.

Discussion

The findings demonstrated that an effective and efficient pilot outreach program had been established. However additional measures were needed to address risks to sustainability of the service and its expansion. To ensure the ongoing quality of the service experienced by both service users and staff, additional planning, and

Table 5.6 Extracts from the observation of the live online service between the outreach worker and service users

Example of STI query	
Online query	What are the symptoms of chlamydia or gonorrhea?
Outreach worker response	A lot of the time, there are no symptoms of these STI's, particularly in the throat. However some people experience burning when peeing, itching and discharge. There is a full explanation of all STI's on the Man2Man website at www.man2man.ie
Example of HIV testing query	
Online query	Hi. Is the immediate HV test thing finished?
Outreach worker response	Know Now rapid HIV testing is still available in all the venues quoted on their website www.knownow.ie GMHS also offer a rapid test at their Monday quick clinic
Example of a sexual behavior query	
Online query	Hello. Is oral sex safe?
Outreach worker response	Using a condom for oral sex can reduce the risk of STIs. Also getting tested regularly for STIs is a good idea if you don't use condoms

resourcing in terms of governance, administrative structures, staffing, and systems were required. This included the recommendation for a stated logic model, the ongoing development of structures for evaluation and monitoring and adequate resourcing of staff.

Case Study 5.2: The Yale Community Healthcare Van Providing Targeted Mobile Outreach Services

Introduction

The Yale University community healthcare van is a mobile medical clinic that serves vulnerable populations in New Haven, Connecticut, United States. New Haven is a small coastal city with a population of approximately 140,000. While it is known for its university, it also has a poverty rate of almost 25% (United States Census Bureau, 2022). The mobile van service was established in 1993 as part of the Yale AIDs program to address a need within the poorest neighborhoods impacted by HIV/AIDS, drug use, homelessness, and mental illness. Its aim is to provide a service but also to link patients to medical and social services. A picture of the van is provided in Fig. 5.1. The management of the van is directed by an advanced nurse practitioner assisted by a team of healthcare professionals and outreach workers.

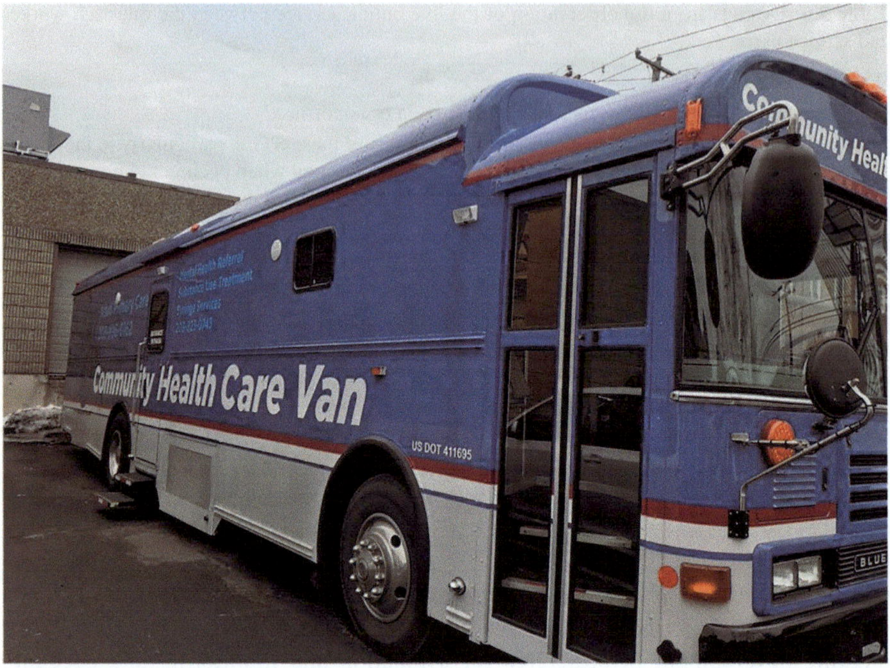

Fig. 5.1 YALE community healthcare van. (Source: C. Comiskey, personal collection)

Methods

To assess patterns of the vans usage and to identify populations who were relying on this non-traditional healthcare, Gibson et al. (2017) conducted a retrospective analysis of the van's visitation records.

Results

The study explored a total of 29,728 visitation records. These visits involved a total of 8415 unique clients. Clients receiving buprenorphine had the highest number of visits with an average of two visits per person per year. Further analysis revealed that being foreign born, a person who injected drugs and having hypertension were factors which increased visits.

Discussion

This study noted that as universal health insurance coverage increases, services such as the mobile van service will continue to play an important role in assisting entry into continuous care for vulnerable urban populations. Building on the vans foundations of addressing unmet needs during healthcare crises such as the 1990s HIV/AIDs epidemic, further details on how the service adapted during the COVID-19 pandemic are provided by Rosenberg et al. (2022).

References

Babor, T. F., Caulkins, J. P., Edwards, G., Fischer, B., Foxcroft, D. R., Humphreys, K., Obot, I. S., Rehm, J., & Reuter, P. (2010). *Drug policy and the public good*. Oxford University Press.

Barker, S. F., Best, D., Manning, V., Savic, M., Lubman, D. I., & Rush, B. (2016). A tiered model of substance use severity and life complexity: Potential for application to needs-based planning. *Substance Abuse, 37*(4), 526–533.

Cohen, J. (1992). A power primer. *Psychological Bulletin*, 112(1), 155–159. Retrieved November 23, 2023, from https://www2.psych.ubc.ca/~schaller/528Readings/Cohen1992.pdf

Comiskey, C., & Dempsey, O. (2013). 18 Analysing data from small and large samples and non-normal and normal distributions. *Quantitative Health Research: Issues And Methods: Issues and Methods, 348*.

Comiskey, C. M., & Snel, A. (2016). Using client's routine urinalysis records from multiple treatment systems to model 5-year opioid substitution treatment outcomes. *Substance Use & Misuse, 51*(4), 498–507.

Comiskey, C., Kelly, P., Leckey, Y., McCullough, L., O'Dúill, B., Stapleton, R., & White, E. (2009). *The ROSIE study: Drug treatment outcomes in Ireland*. Stationery Office.

Comiskey, C. M., O'Sullivan, K., Quirke, M. B., Wynne, C., Kelly, P., & McGilloway, S. (2012). *Evaluation of the effectiveness of the childhood development initiative's healthy schools programme* (ISBN: 978-0-9570232-4-6). https://www.cdi.ie/wp-content/uploads/2016/11/CDI-HSP-Report-12.11-web.pdf

Comiskey, C. M., McCarthy, E. M., Swithenbank, Z., & Hay, G. (2023). *Evaluating treatment outcomes from drug policies and practices, chapter 8 in evaluating the impact of laws regulating illicit drugs on health and society*. Bentham Science Publishers Pte. Ltd.

Cox, G., & Comiskey, C. (2007). Characteristics of opiate users presenting for a new treatment episode: Baseline data from the national drug treatment outcome study in Ireland (ROSIE). *Drugs: Education, Prevention and Policy, 14*(3), 217–230.

Darke, S., Ross, J., Teesson, M., Ali, R., Cooke, R., Ritter, A., & Lynskey, M. (2005). Factors associated with 12 months continuous heroin abstinence: Findings from the Australian Treatment Outcome Study (ATOS). *Journal of Substance Abuse Treatment, 28*(3), 255–263.

EMIS. (2019). *The EMIS Network. EMIS-2017—The European men-who-have-sex-with-men internet survey*. Key findings from 50 countries. Retrieved November 22, 2023, from https://www.ecdc.europa.eu/en/publications-data/emis-2017-european-men-who-have-sex-men-internet-survey

Gibson, B. A., Morano, J. P., Walton, M. R., Marcus, R., Zelenev, A., Bruce, R. D., & Altice, F. L. (2017). Innovative Program Delivery and Determinants of Frequent Visitation to a Mobile Medical Clinic in an Urban Setting. *Journal of health care for the poor and underserved, 28*(2), 643–662. https://doi.org/10.1353/hpu.2017.0065

Gossop, M., Marsden, J., Stewart, D., & Rolfe, A. (2000). Patterns of drinking and drinking outcomes among drug misusers. 1-year follow-up results. *Journal of Substance Abuse Treatment, 19*(1), 45–50. http://ovidsp.ovid.com/ovidweb.cgi?T=JS&PAGE=reference&D=med4&NEWS=N&AN=10867300

Healthy Ireland. (2015). *National sexual health strategy 2015–2020*. Retrieved November 22, 2023, from https://assets.gov.ie/7562/e5a5ac26eb22405aaf6538656564690a.pdf

McKeganey, N., Bloor, M., Robertson, M., Neale, J., & MacDougall, J. (2006). Abstinence and drug abuse treatment: results from the drug outcome research in Scotland study. *Drugs: Education, Prevention and Policy, 13*(6), 537–550.

Mosel, S. (2023). *Levels of Care for Addiction Treatment*. Retrieved 21 November 2023, from americanaddictioncenters.org

National Treatment Agency. (2002). *Models of care for treatment of adult drug misusers. Available as Part 1: Summary for Commissioners and Managers Responsible for Implementation, and Part 2:* Full Reference Report.

National Treatment Agency for Substance Misuse. (2006). *Models of care for treatment of adult drug misusers: Update 2006*. Retrieved November 21, 2023, from https://www.drugsandalcohol.ie/20325/1/nta_modelsofcare_update_2006.pdf

NIDA. (2012). *Principles of drug addiction treatment: A research-based guide*. Retrieved November 20, 2023, from https://www.drugabuse.gov/sites/default/files/podat_1.pdf

Rosenberg, J., Sude, L., Budge, M., León-Martínez, D., Fenick, A., Altice, F. L., & Sharifi, M. (2022). Rapid deployment of a mobile medical clinic during the COVID-19 pandemic: Assessment of dyadic maternal-child care. *Maternal Child Health Journal, 26*(9), 1762–1778. https://doi.org/10.1007/s10995-022-03483-6

Rush, B. (2010). Tiered frameworks for planning substance use ser-vice delivery systems: Origins and key principles. *Nordic Studies on Alcohol and Drugs*, 27(6), 617–636. Retrieved November 21, 2023, from https://journals.sagepub.com/doi/pdf/10.1177/145507251002700607

Rush, B., & Furlong, A. (2020). *Rapid access models for substance use services: A rapid review*. Retrieved November 20, 2023, from https://www.ccsa.ca/sites/default/files/2020-10/CCSA-Rapid-Access-Models-Substance-Use-Services-Rapid-Review-Report-2020-en.pdf

Rush, B., Tremblay, J., Fougere, C., Behrooz, R. C., Perez, W., & Fineczko, J. (2014). *Development of a needs-based planning model for substance use services and supports in Canada: Final report 2010–2014*. Retrieved November 21, 2023, from https://doi.org/10.13140/RG.2.2.32719.59046

Rush, B., Tremblay, J., & Brown, D. (2019). Development of a needs-based planning model to estimate required capacity of a substance use treatment system. Supplement 18, 51–63. Retrieved November 21, 2023, from https://www.jsad.com/doi/10.15288/jsads.2019.s18.51

Simpson, D. D. (2003). Introduction to 5-year followup treatment outcome studies. *Journal of Substance Abuse Treatment, 25*(3), 123–124.

WHO and UNODC. (2020). *International standards for the treatment of drug use disorders: Revised edition incorporating results of field-testing*. Retrieved November 20, 2023, from https://www.unodc.org/documents/drug-prevention-and-treatment/UNODC-WHO_International_Standards_Treatment_Drug_Use_Disorders_April_2020.pdf

United States Census Bureau. (2022). *QuickFacts New Haven city, Connecticut*. Retrieved 24 November 2023, from https://www.census.gov/quickfacts/fact/table/newhavencityconnecticut/POP060210

Chapter 6
Disaster Preparedness, Rapid Assessment, Response, Recovery, and Foresight: Responding to Unplanned Events and Emerging Threats

Setting the Scene

Oleksander navigates a bomb-shelled northern Ukrainian city between air raid sirens. He is on his way to the clinic to collect methadone for his opioid use disorder... 3 days earlier he sent his wife and children to Lviv for safety and has been living with 20 other men in the basement of his building, which doubles as a bomb shelter...Yesterday, his doctor texted him a 30-min window to pick up his methadone, when emergency sirens are less common... Even though Ukraine's Ministry of Health has just released new guidance allowing for a 30-day supply, his doctor is reluctant because he needs to keep enough for his other patients... Extract from Altice et al. (2022, p. e482)

Introduction

While disasters can occur naturally such as earthquakes, floods, tornadoes, hurricanes, wildfires, mudslides, or drought; they can also be caused by humans with mass shootings or mass street violence, chemical spills, and targeted chemical warfare or terrorist attacks. Indeed, they can also be the consequence of poor economic policies or governance infrastructure, such as bank failures, wide scale corruption with vested interests and national cyberattacks. It is widely recognized that preparing for, responding to, and recovering from disasters and traumatic events is essential to the behavioral health of individuals and communities (SAMHSA, 2023).

C. Comiskey, *Addiction Research and Evaluation*, Advances in Mental Health and Addiction, https://doi.org/10.1007/978-3-031-65917-1_6

The Sendai Framework for Disaster Risk Reduction 2015–2030

This framework is a blueprint for making communities safer and more resilient. The framework provides Member States with concrete actions to protect development gains from the risks posed by disasters. The United Nations Office for Disaster Risk Reduction (UNDRR) supports the implementation, follow-up, and review of the Sendai Framework and coordinates actions within the UN system around disaster risk reduction (UNDRR, 2023).

The framework is the outcome of stakeholder consultations and inter-governmental negotiations which were supported by the UNDRR. It is designed to be compatible with the Paris Agreement on Climate Change, the Addis Ababa Action Agenda on Financing for Development, the New Urban Agenda, and the Sustainable Development Goals (UNDRR, 2023).

The Sendai Framework chart has the stated goal to:

Prevent new and reduce existing disaster risk through the implementation of integrated and inclusive economic, structural, legal, social, health, cultural, educational, environmental, technological, political, and institutional measures that prevent and reduce hazard exposure and vulnerability to disaster, increase preparedness for response and recovery, and thus strengthen resilience (UNDRR, 2023).

The priority areas of the Sendai Framework are provided in Table 6.1.

Managing Risk in a Work Environment

Within employment, health and safety legislation mandates employers and service providers to manage risk and risk assessment in work environments. The five simple steps to manage risk are provided in Table 6.2.

When a disaster or an adverse unexpected advent is experienced, many people exhibit resilience, that is, the ability to cope with adversity and endure difficult situations. Resilience in disaster recovery is to be expected and it is not extraordinary, as people are generally resilient. However, some people will exhibit additional stress following a disaster and this is important to address. This additional stress may exacerbate existing mental health or substance use problems. It is important to

Table 6.1 The priority areas of the United Nations, Sendai Framework for Disaster Risk Reduction 2015–2030

Priority areas of the United Nations
Understanding disaster risk
Strengthening disaster risk governance in order to manage risk
Invest in disaster risk reduction for resilience
Enhance disaster preparedness for effective responses and importantly to "build Back better" in recovery

Table 6.2 The five steps for managing risk in a work environment (Health and Safety Executive, 2023)

Five steps for managing risk in a work environment	
1. Identify hazards	Review the workplace, remembering workplace users of all levels of ability
2. Assess the risks	Decide how likely it is that someone could be harmed and how serious it could be
3. Control the risks	Review what is already in place and seek to eliminate the hazard fully if possible or else reduce it
4. Record your findings	Depending on your local legislation you may be required to record and report on your risk assessment findings and mitigation steps
5. Review the controls	Review your controls to ensure they are still effective or review if you have changes in staffing, equipment or processes

monitor the physical and emotional health of those affected as well as those people who are responding to the needs of others.

The Rapid Assessment and Response (RAR) Approach

As public health issues can emerge and change rapidly over time many of the public and behavioral health issues will require a quicker response than traditional scientific research allows for. This has led to the development of what is known as Rapid Assessment approaches. One of the key documents detailing Rapid Assessment and Response (RAR) guidelines were developed by WHO and UNAIDS (WHO, 1998). These were further developed within Europe and the European Drug Agency (EMCDDA, 2004), formerly the European Monitoring Centre for Drugs and Drug Addiction.

The EMCDDA explains that RAR approaches help with gathering information on needs quickly and within varying cultural settings. It is particularly useful for selective prevention with specific groups at risk. Braam and Varbraeck (2017) have built upon these earlier guidelines and have provided a RAR manual for substance use and addiction.

The RAR approach to gathering evidence for interventions to address alcohol and the use of other substances among people displaced by conflict has been studied (Ezard et al., 2011). Alcohol use in Columbia, khat chewing in Somalia, benzodiazepines use in Bosnia-Herzegovina, opiates in Afghanistan and Pakistan and a range of other substances have been highlighted among people impacted by wars and conflicts, according to Ezard et al. (2011).

More recently within Ukraine the challenging of accessing methadone for opiate use disorder during the war has been highlighted (Altice et al., 2022). Some treatment centers had to reduce doses provided to individuals to enable supplies to last longer. Many other centers did not know if supplies would be replenished. As a consequence of the war, there was a fear that people experiencing sudden withdrawal symptoms would be at a greater risk of relapsing to possibly injecting opioids, risking overdosing and transmission of blood borne viruses such a HIV and Hepatitis C.

Ezard et al. (2011) studied six rapid assessments of alcohol and other substance use in populations displaced by conflict. The sources of data were individual and group interviews conducted with a culturally representative sample of community members and service providers. The authors found that limited access to services, including health services, and exclusion from relevant host population programs, could exacerbate the harmful consequences of the alcohol and substance use. They also stated that the six studies showed the feasibility and value in conducting rapid assessments and the need for more experience in delivering effective interventions under these circumstances.

The Theory of Rapid Assessment and Response

The foundations of RAR are within applied anthropology, sociology, epidemiology, and evaluation research methods (WHO, 1998). Braam and Varbraeck (2017) however, state that the approach has also been used in the past to identify new markets for commercial products. The rapid outbreak of HIV/AIDs globally in the late decades of the twentieth century was the rationale for developing scientific-based methods that could respond to urgent public and behavioral health dual challenges of infection and intravenous drug use in a pragmatic yet evidenced informed way.

Since the promotion of the method for HIV/AIDs research, it has been tested and used in diverse populations and settings, as seen by Ezard et al. (2011) among people experiencing conflict; Dupont et al. (2015) among young populations using cannabis; and Comiskey et al. (2012) using RAR approaches to guide the reduction of drug services in times of economic crises.

RAR a fast and cost-effective approach which uses several data collection methods including interviews, focus groups and audit and observation with culturally and demographically appropriate groups in relation to the problem being addressed. It helps responders to understand and explore an emerging phenomenon rather than providing quantifiable evidence. Cross-checking, triangulating, weighing and eventually funneling the evidence from a wide range of backgrounds is a key component of the approach. The network of collaborators consulted can also be harnessed to devise appropriate responses and interventions for the setting. As Braam and Varbraeck (2017) state, RAR is a pragmatic approach focusing on adequacy rather than on scientific evidence.

Features of Rapid Assessment

The key features of RAR are provided by WHO (1998) and are adapted and summarized in Table 6.3 within the context of substance use.

Foresight Exercises

The use of foresight exercises is not new, and the approaches have been used in the private business section since the 1970s (EMCDDA, 2022). Since the emergence of the COVID-19 global pandemic, the awareness of the need for these exercises has become more obvious. Indeed, a potential global pandemic was itself predicted within a futures exercise where it was stated, "In many ways, a global pandemic has to be seen as a greater threat to us than nuclear terrorism and global warming combined" (Future Agenda, 2011, p. 63). While both global terrorisms, be it bioterrorism or nuclear and global warming, are still major threats to the planet and its people, the global threat of a pandemic has been realized as predicted.

Futures exercises and foresight have also been used by the United Nations in efforts to improve multi-year planning for the UN Development Assistance Framework and the Sustainable Development Goals implementation (UN Sustainable Development Group, 2016). Finally, the WHO have recognized the importance of foresight within global public health and have invested in developing training in this (WHO, 2022).

The EMCDDA (2022) have used the approach to develop scenarios for the future of European drug monitoring and responses. The key principle of foresight is for organizations and individuals to behave proactively rather than reactively, to identify and anticipate change and to be prepared with varying options should they be needed. The approach involves creating potential scenarios of possibilities rather than predictions or forecasts and the emphasis is on developing flexible strategies that can adapt and be applied to several possible futures. The approach uses less rigorous scientific conventional prediction methods but rather it is based on specialist and novel methods.

Future Agenda (2011) provides a good schematic to explain the relationships between insight, trends, and foresight and Fig. 6.1 reflects this.

In the work of the EMCDDA (2022), trends analysis is one of the key methodologies they suggest is used as a building block within substance use services. Examples of the typical steps of a trend analysis is provided in Fig. 6.2 based on the EMCDDA work. Within step 2, it is important to check for any blind spots. This is done to make sure nothing is missed or overlooked. That no potentially critical high impact developments have been missed. Within step 3, trends that are more relevant to the topic or the organization are prioritized. In step 4 when analyzing implications respective option for action today can be explored.

Table 6.3 Ten key features of rapid assessment

Ten key features of rapid assessment	
Speed	As was seen with the emergence of HIV/AIDs in the twentieth century, the impact of wars in the twenty-first century and the rise of the use of technology in drug markets and drug products. New drugs, new patterns of sale and new infections can emerge rapidly and require a response that conventional research cannot address in a prompt timeframe
Cost effectiveness	RAR research techniques have a high output of information in relation to the input of research effort. Comiskey et al. (2012) used RAR to evaluate 30 drug services in three months given pending budget cut back decisions. There is a preference for cheaper sources of data collection
Exploitation of data	Existing data resources that are available are used in perhaps new ways. Costly surveys are only used if no existing data is available or adequate to include within the triangulation
Use of multiple indicators and data sources	Several varying sources of data are used as a single source cannot encompass all aspects of the problem. An overview is constructed from the varying data sources
An investigative orientation	As in many cultural settings, substance use may be very hidden and linked with stigma. RAR researchers need to adopt a thorough and constant cross-checking of data to identify any hidden biases in the information. An example of such hidden data may be mothers accessing substance use services but are also experiencing domestic abuse in the form of economic abuse. Or men who use substances and pay for sex with men and are not using condoms
Inductive approach	RAR researchers when faced with a new and emerging risk should use an inductive approach to building their findings. Inductive analysis works by establishing initial descriptions and hypotheses about the problem, and refining these in the light of further evidence that leads to confirmation, modification or rejection of the descriptions and hypotheses according to WHO (1998)
Relevance to interventions and decision-making	A RAR is not a product, rather it allows you to develop an intervention or make difficult decisions on resources and targets of responses to needs identified. A RAR is judged not on its scientific rigor but rather on its utility in progressing to an informed response to the disaster, risk and need identified
RAR investigation is at several levels	Drug problems may be developing and may be linked beyond the individual and community levels. Economic, social, cultural, religious, political, and historical contexts are important to consider
Consultation and community involvement	People who use drugs and their families, peers or communities are important to involve ensuring a wide range of voices are considered. These groups are also essential to ensure any solutions proposed are feasible and practical. For example, if a new needle exchange is to be introduced where should it be located? Mothers with young children may not be able to travel or older rural dwellers may not have access to transport. Would a mobile bus service be more appropriate?
The principle of adequacy as opposed to scientific perfection	Rigor, reliability, and validity are obtained through cross-checking of data sources, triangulation and the inclusivity and diversity of collaborators. Triangulation and inductive reasoning to establish findings from multiple data sources are also discussed by Braun and Clarke (2006) if more details on these terms are needed

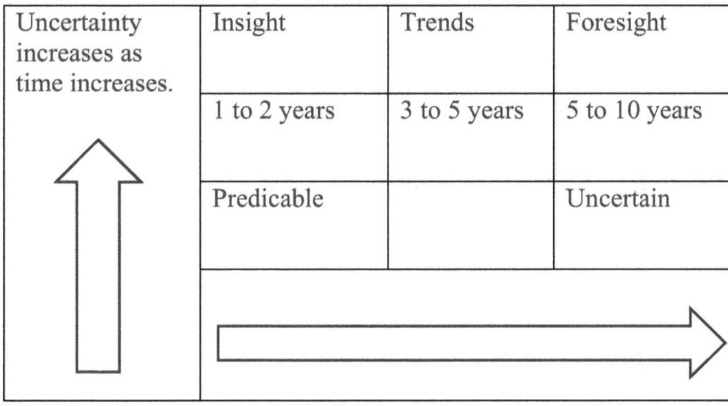

Fig. 6.1 The relationship between insight, trends, and foresight. Adapted from Future Agenda (2011)

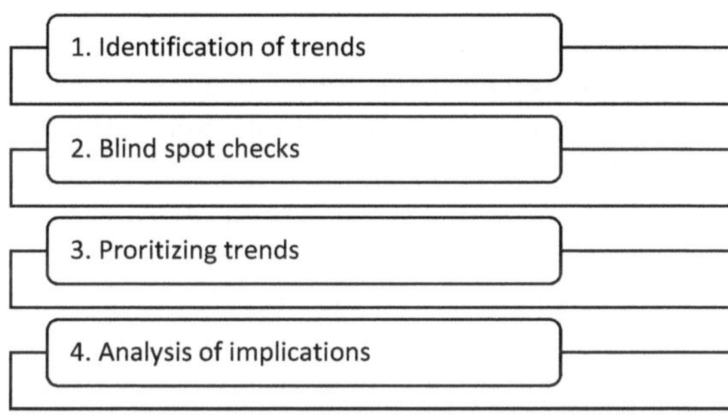

Fig. 6.2 The four steps involved in a trend analysis. (Adapted from EMCDDA, 2022)

Approaches other than trend analysis which can be used and should be combined with the trend scanning is scenario development, Delphi surveys, and approaches that look at potential disruptions or wild cards. The principle of a 360-degree view is essential when conducting this exercise. The 360-degree view involves scanning not just the areas of focus of one's organization but a variety of other areas. The so called "STEEP" approach of looking at Social, Technological, Economic, Environmental, and Political aspects can be used to help identify any blind spots in the exercise.

Future Agenda (2011) which was based on a broader remit used not just trend analysis but extensive global consultation both online and face-to-face workshops with contributors who included experts and others working across these five aspects of the STEEP approach.

To conclude according to SAMHSA (2016), the key to disaster response is to be prepared in advance by conducting foresight and preparedness exercises as opposed to responding after the event. While one can never be fully prepared, foresight can help prepare communities, service providers, practitioners, and policy makers.

Two case studies addressing rapid assessment and response and foresight are described below for additional learning. Due to their rapid response to unfolding emergencies, RAR initiatives can sometimes be controversial as these two examples in very different settings, both geographically and economically illustrate.

Case Study 6.1a: Rapid Assessment and Response: Responding to a City's Fentanyl Crisis

Introduction

Kerr et al. (2017) have chartered the background and history to the first supervised injection facilities in Canada. In response to HIV and overdose epidemics in the mid-1990s a group of advocates led by people who used drugs with a group of health professionals opened the first unsanctioned safe injection site in Vancouver in 1995. Anecdotally it was reported that sign-in sheets collected at the site recorded over 100 people each night and nurses visited the site to provide support. The site was eventually shut down after a year.

A safe injection site or safe injection facility (SIF) also known as a supervised consumption site or an overdose prevention site, is a safe space where trained staff can monitor people who use illicit drugs and help prevent harm, disease transmission and reduce overdoses and deaths. They benefit communities and individuals as they connect people who use drugs to appropriate health or social services. They bring stability to communities by improving public order and reducing drug consumption on the streets (Vancouver Coastal Health, 2023).

From the first unsanctioned site in 1995, it took until 2003 for the first official site to open. This site was built by a nongovernmental organization in a vacant building without approval and it simply opened. Prior to this Health Canada had released its SIF guideline document and shortly afterwards this first SIF location called Insite was sanctioned. Insite was allowed to open as a pilot study and had to be rigorously evaluated (Kerr et al., 2006). Progress in developing further sites was slow and challenging both legally and socially. As the number of deaths due to fentanyl overdoses increased the need for a more rapid response was urgently needed.

Method

In 2016, it was reported by Vancouver Coastal Health that of 332 drug checks performed by Insite in a 2-month period between July seventh to September eighth, 80% of all drugs tested and 85% of heroin samples tested contained fentanyl (Lupick, 2016a). During this time long lines were forming at sanctioned SIFs and they could not meet demand. In response, in September 2016, two advocates and community organizers Sarah Blyth and Ann Livingston decided to set up a tent and open an unsanctioned site on a back alley in Vancouver where people were using drugs. The tent was established in response to the rise in overdoses deaths due to the fentanyl contamination. This rapid response was built upon years of former evidence on the role and efficacy of SIFs and the newly emerging evidence of the link between the rise in deaths among people who use drugs and fentanyl. Within the alley-based tent, supplies of syringes, rubber bands, and alcohol swabs were readily available. At that time there were also a small number of naloxone injections available to reverse overdoses on sites. Within 2 months following what Blyth described as "the most horrible week ever," a further tent was set up by Blyth and Livingston to start a second unsanctioned supervised injection site (Lupick, 2016b).

Discussion

Other temporary unsanctioned safe injecting facilities began to emerge across Canada in response to the fentanyl crisis. These sites provided lower levels of support than Insite, they were used frequently and prevented many deaths. As federal (national) approval was required to open a sanctioned SIF, the regions health minister instructed the local health authorities to establish what became known as Overdose Prevention Sites (OPS). The sites operated with less levels of service than Insite and had a different service design. Within a few days of this instruction an OPS was opened at VANDU, a peer-led organization supporting people who use drugs (Kerr et al., 2017). Furthermore, the three women, Sarah Blyth, Ann Livingston, and Chris Ewart, responsible for setting up the first tent were subsequently recognized for their life saving yet controversial efforts and were awarded the first-ever British Columbia, Civil Liberties Association (BCCLA) Jennifer Prosser Wade Award for Courage: Where truth speaks to power (Lupick, 2017).

Case Study 6.1b: Rapid Assessment and Response: Responding to an Economic Crisis in Rural Drug Services

Introduction

Within Ireland, substance misuse services are organized and funded on both a national and a regional basis. Following a sudden economic crash in 2008, post the so called "Celtic Tiger" funding for regional substance use services were severely cut. The Celtic Tiger was experienced between 1995 and 2007 and was the popular name for an economic boom. The Irish economy grew at an average rate of 9.4% during this period. The term was intended to reflect the Four Asian Tigers, the nations of Singapore, Hong Kong, Taiwan, and South Korea. Each of these countries also experienced very rapid economic growth rates more than 7% a year between the mid-1950s, for Hong Kong and the early 1960s for the other three countries (Peters, 2021).

Given the challenges with continuing funding for regional drug services, one locality sought to base their funding decisions on the service performance in relation to the needs of their local population. The region commissioned research to:

1. Undertake a needs assessment with regards to the scale and nature of substance use in the region.
2. Conduct an evaluation of the effectiveness and efficiency of resource use in 30 of the drug projects it was funding.
3. Given the needs assessment, the review of the projects funded and the national drug strategy, develop a road map for future substance use services in the region.

These three would then be used by the regional authorities to assist their decision-making on the necessary cutbacks.

Methods

Given the scale of the task and the speed within which decisions had to be made a Rapid Assessment and Response was undertaken with a timescale of 3 months (Comiskey et al., 2012).

To address the first objective, outputs from a range of existing data bases were requested. This included outputs from three national drug indicators. The treatment demand indicator, which provided data on all drug and alcohol treatments in the region. The general population survey on drug use, which was an indicator of prevalence. The third indicator was the problem drug use indicator, which provided details on the number estimated to be using opiates or cocaine in the region. This was also accessed. These indicators provided objective measures of need.

To provide subjective indicators of need an open-ended needs assessment questionnaire was administered to each service. This formed the basis of a subjective, prospective needs analysis. A one-to-one interview with one key informant within each of the 30 services was conducted. Data from all these sources was then triangulated to provide an assessment of need.

To address the second objective, the one-to-one interviews also addressed the aims and objective of the service as described in their service plan and a discussion on this. Each service also completed a template on service provision. A review of the services financial monitoring against their service agreements aims and objectives was also conducted. Follow-up consultations by e-mail and phone were also conducted to fill in any gaps in the information and clarify any information that was not clear. Finally, a consultation with other regional stakeholders for their views was undertaken. A copy of the template for assessing services is provided in Table 6.4.

To develop the road map for the region in line with the national strategy a detailed triangulation of findings was conducted by the full team. Triangulation according to WHO (1998) is the continual process of collecting and cross-checking information.

Table 6.4 Template for a service evaluation. (Adapted from Comiskey et al., 2012)

Project number: xxx Funding received: € xxx Target group (from service level agreement): xxx Description of the project: xxx Aims and objectives of the regional funding: xxx		
Efficiency	**Evidence examples**	**Attached Score 1 = Yes, 0 = No**
(a) Provided evidence of how service publicizes hours of operation and the location of service	Leaflets, Web advertising, etc.	
(b) Provided evidence of the accessibility criteria that is available to (i) services referring to the project, (ii) individuals that wish to self-refer	List of criteria available to services	
(c) Had a documented service specification that detailed—The aims and objectives of the outreach service, the target group, and working methods	Documentary evidence	
(d) Carries out a needs assessment with each client	Client files	
(e) Goals and/or referrals set out in assessments and agreed by both service user and service provider	Client files	
(f) Information is provided to service users in relation to other services that they can access	Leaflets, service lists/ staff interview	
(g) Written protocols around coordinated working processes between service and other services and agencies in relation to service users	Policies/procedures	
(h) Demonstrated how service users are supported in accessing other services where relevant	Client files/staff interview	
Evaluation of efficiencies: xxx Observations from the monitoring data: xxx Summary and conclusions: xxx Service response to evaluation (150 words): xxx		

Using a combination of different methods and different data sources, a cross-check is carried out to check for contradictions, conflicts, or consensus between data sources.

Results

Overall, the Rapid Assessment and Response found that not all services were meeting the emerging needs that had been identified in the RAR. Services lacked administrative support to fulfil their objectives and funding needed to be redirected to priority areas. The RAR approach was found to be very useful for aiding policy and budgetary conditions in times of unexpected financial crisis and imminent and stringent cutbacks. Detailed findings are provided by Comiskey et al. (2012) and an extract from the road map is provided in Table 6.5. Understandably findings were very sensitive.

Table 6.5 An extract from the roadmap for service priority following a RAR exercise in a rural region. (Extracted from Comiskey et al., 2012)

Project number	Category	Priority one
P-5	Treatment	Continue to fund
P-10	Family support/ prevention	Continue to fund
P-11	Family support/ prevention	Continue to fund
P-12	Treatment	Continue to fund
P-15	Family support/ prevention	Continue to fund
P-18	Prevention	Continue to fund
P-23	Treatment	Continue to fund
P-24	Treatment	Continue to fund
P-28	Family support	Continue to fund
P-26	Treatment	Continue to fund
P-21	Treatment	Continue to fund. Monitoring data appears to show effectiveness however further evidence of efficiencies should be demonstrated to funder
P-3	Family support	Continue to fund but review use of staff capacity
P-32	Treatment	Continue to fund—However the project needs to demonstrate greater efficiencies and refinement of target groups
Project number	**Category**	**Priority two**
P-2	Rehabilitation	Continue to fund but review amount in context of service provision to region
P-27	Rehabilitation	Continue to fund but review amount and refine monitoring data
P-34	Rehabilitation	Continue to fund—But review amount/target group
Project number	**Category**	**Priority three**
P-1	Rehabilitation	Suspend funding. The evaluation team recognizes the need for family support services. However residential respite is considered to be cost intensive in the context of the need to cut back spending
P-4	Prevention	Suspend funding based on the evaluation. This project was set up as a pilot. However, it must be recognized that the area has a higher number of people using drugs
P-6	Prevention	Suspension on funding to continue. However, the evaluation acknowledges that the project did attempt to target a group of high-risk young people in need
P-7	Prevention	Suspension of funding to continue

Discussion

Findings were communicated at an open meeting with all service providers invited. They were presented simultaneously, in an anonymized manner where each service provider would know only their own service number. While decisions for the local regional funder were difficult it was appreciated by service providers that decisions were evidence informed, based on an objective assessment of the needs of the region and priorities were identified independently and without any conflicts of interest.

Case Study 6.2: Using a Foresight "Futures Study" to Explore Drug Research Priorities Within the European Union

Introduction

As the European drug situation and drug markets become increasingly diverse, complex, and dynamic the European Monitoring Centre for Drugs and Drug Addiction sought to strengthen its strategic planning with the piloting of a foresight approach and a futures exercise focusing on its drug monitoring role in Europe (EMCDDA, 2023). The exercise was subsequently expanded and built upon to pilot the identification of drug research priorities for the region. Prior to this pilot study, drug research priorities were identified by the agency's independent Scientific Committee. This committee of independently appointed experts from across Europe had a legal mandate to advise annually on the agency's program of work and to conduct risk assessments for new psychoactive drugs when requested.

The Scientific Committee were also invited on an annual basis to address Europe's Horizontal Working Party on Drugs in Brussels. The group was known as the HDG, the Horizontal Drugs Group (HDG) and the Scientific Committee presented the annual dialogue on drug research priorities to them. The HDG was established in 1997 and was responsible for leading and managing the Council's work on drugs. Their work is focused on three cross-cutting themes: coordination, international cooperation, and research, monitoring and evaluation (European Council of the European Union, 2024).

In 2021, the Scientific Committee drafted a position paper on extending the EMCDDA's monitoring and reporting framework to cover the substance misuse topic and its consequences for European policies and responses in a more holistic manner. This was presented at the HDG, emphasizing the importance of adopting a more holistic, conceptual framework of polydrug use in research to underpin more effective evidence-based policy, prevention, and practice.

Methods

To assist with identifying the research priorities of the future, the EMCDDA extended the learning from their original futures exercise and piloted the approach a second time. The second pilot study consisted of a Delphi study with 25 theses topics based on findings form the first futures exercise. Participants from a range of relevant stakeholders including the Scientific Committee and relevant EMCDDA staff were asked to rate these for impact, certainty, and earliest time to maturity.

Results

The original study identified five megatrends as the most significant for driving change in the drugs area. A megatrend is defined as long-term driving force that is globally observable now and will most likely significantly influence the future in many different fields. Megatrends are larger than the power of individual organizations and often nation states as well.

The five megatrends were:

1. Accelerating technological change and hyperconnectivity.
2. Diversifying inequalities.
3. Shifting health challenges.
4. Population changes.
5. Climate change and environmental degradation.

Four possible emerging trends were identified. Emerging trends are considered relatively strong and visible, or new developments that are being observed within some sources and with some evidence.

The emerging trends were:

1. A shift in drug policy and drug laws.
2. A shift in the discourse of addiction.
3. A shift in drug production.
4. A shift in drug services.

In terms of the research priority findings, results are provided in Table 6.6. Earliest time to maturity was not considered a forecast but rather after a certain date specified, it may already be too late to react. The time was within the next 4–10 years.

Additional priorities identified within comments by the Scientific Committee outside of the Delphi theses reflected ongoing concerns which needed to be addressed.

These additional current priorities were:

- Psychiatric comorbidity in people who use drugs: detection and treatment.
- Social determinants of health in access to commodities and treatment.
- The role of stigma and inaccessibility to services for certain communities.

Table 6.6 Findings from the Delphi futures exercise on drug research priorities as conducted in 2021 by the EMCDDA with its independent Scientific Committee. (Extracted from the presentation by Comiskey to the HDG in Brussels on October 25th 2022)

Consensus where the earliest effects would be seen:
The spread of polydrug use, including nonmedical use of medicines (thesis 20)
Innovations in drug distribution (thesis 5)
Increasing instability in Europe's neighboring regions (thesis 15)
Theses rated as most significant for the drugs field over the next ten years by certainty and impact
Thesis 12: Cannabis policies will further evolve and commercialization of legal cannabis will increase
Thesis 11: Further increase in digitalization in the drug field will impact security and/or health responses
Thesis 20: The prevalence of polydrug use, including the importance of the nonmedical use of medicines will increase
Thesis 4: Production of synthetic drugs such as high potency products, new psychoactive substances and fake medicines will increase

- The importance of upholding a harm reduction philosophy.
- Research the determinants of drug use for prevention policies.
- Focus on effective, tailored prevention measures.
- Lack of training and workforce in addictions services.
- Polydrug use, mainly alcohol and tobacco.

Discussion

Following the identification of the research priorities by the Scientific Committee through the foresight exercise and the Delphi approach it was agreed by the committee that the exercise was extremely useful and could be used again after this initial pilot study. The committee welcomed the approach and the findings and thought it would be an appropriate way forward for the new mandate of the EMCDDA. This new mandate would change to the European Drugs Agency (EUDA). This was particularly relevant as the new agency under Article 21 of its foundation was tasked with,

> *assisting the Commission and the Member States in identifying key research themes, drawing up and implementing the Union framework programmes for research and innovation activities.*

Furthermore, reviewing with hindsight, the findings on what were deemed to be the earliest effects, it is validating of the exercise to note that in 2021 prior to the initiation of Russian/Ukraine war in February 2022 and the Israel and Gaza conflict in October 2023 it was stated that increasing instability in Europe's neighboring regions would influence the drugs situation in Europe.

References

Altice, F. L., Bromberg, D. J., Dvoriak, S., Meteliuk, A., Pykalo, I., Islam, Z., Azbel, L., & Madden, L. M. (2022). Extending a lifeline to people with HIV and opioid use disorder during the war in Ukraine. *The Lancet Public Health, 7*(5), e482–e484. https://www.thelancet.com/action/showPdf?pii=S2468-2667%2822%2900083-4

Braam, R., & Varbraeck, H. (2017). *RAR manual substance use and addiction*. Correlation European Harm Reduction Network. Retrieved November 23, 2024, from https://www.correlation-net.org/wp-content/uploads/2018/12/RAR-manual-substance-use-and-addiction.pdf

Braun, V., & Clarke, V. (2006). Using thematic analysis in psychology. *Qualitative Research in Psychology, 3*(2), 77–101. https://doi.org/10.1191/1478088706qp063oa

Comiskey, C. M., O'Sullivan, K., & Milnes, J. (2012). Regional drug user services in times of scarce financial resources: Using a rapid assessment response approach to evaluate, plan, and prioritize essential services. *Substance Use & Misuse, 47*(3), 254–264.

Dupont, H. B., Kaplan, C. D., Braam, R. V., Verbraeck, H. T., & de Vries, N. K. (2015). The application of the rapid assessment and response methodology for cannabis prevention research among youth in The Netherlands. *International Journal of Drug Policy, 26*(8), 731–738.

EMCDDA. (2004). *EMCDDA recommended draft technical tools and guidelines.* Key Epidemiological Indicator: Prevalence of problem drug use (9291681733).

EMCDDA. (2022) *How to run a trends workshop: An EMCDDA foresight toolkit for the drugs field.* Publications Office of the European Union. Available at: https://www.emcdda.europa.eu/publications/manuals-and-guidelines/how-run-trends-workshop-emcdda-foresight-toolkit-drugs-field_en. Accessed 04 June 2024.

EMCDDA. (2023). *The future of drug monitoring in Europe until 2030: A report summarising the findings and lessons learnt from the EMCDDA's 'futures study'*. Available at: https://www.emcdda.europa.eu/publications/technical-reports/future-drug-monitoring-europe-until-2030_en. Accessed 01 December 2023.

European Council of the European Union. (2024). *Horizontal Working Party on Drugs (HDG) – Consilium, European Council of the European Union.* Available at: https://www.consilium.europa.eu/en/council-eu/preparatory-bodies/horizontal-working-party-drugs/. Accessed 04 June 2024.

Ezard, N., Oppenheimer, E., Burton, A., Schilperoord, M., Macdonald, D., Adelekan, M., Sakarati, A., & Van Ommeren, M. (2011). Six rapid assessments of alcohol and other substance use in populations displaced by conflict. *Conflict and Health, 5*, 1–15.

Future Agenda. (2011). *The world in 2020, Oxford 2011.* Retrieved November 29, 2023, from https://www.futureagenda.org/wp-content/uploads/2019/10/Future-Agenda_final-2020.pdf

Kerr, T., Stoltz, J.-A., Tyndall, M., Li, K., Zhang, R., Montaner, J., & Wood, E. (2006). Impact of a medically supervised safer injection facility on community drug use patterns: A before and after study. *BMJ, 332*(7535), 220–222.

Kerr, T., Mitra, S., Kennedy, M. C., & McNeil, R. (2017). Supervised injection facilities in Canada: Past, present, and future. *Harm Reduction Journal, 14*(1), 1–9.

Lupick, T. (2016a). *Cheap and easy: Fentanyl test strips show prom-ise as new tool in B.C.'s struggle with overdose deaths.* Retrieved November 28, 2023, from Cheap and easy: fentanyl test strips show promise as new tool in B.C.'s struggle with overdose deaths | Georgia Straight Vancou-ver's source for arts, culture, and events.

Lupick, T. (2016b). *Downtown Eastside activists offer supervised-injection services for drug users at second unsanctioned tent.* Retrieved November 28, 2023, from https://www.straight.com/news/831541/downtown-eastside-activists-offer-supervised-injection-services-drug-users-second

Lupick, T. (2017). *Downtown Eastside activists to receive BCCLA award for bending the rules to save addicts' lives.* Retrieved November 30, 2023, from https://www.straight.com/news/903571/downtown-eastside-activists-receive-bccla-award-bending-rules-save-addicts-lives

Peters, K. (2021). *Celtic tiger: Definition, history, and how irish economy thrived.* Retrieved December 1, 2023, from Celtic Tiger: Definition, History, and How Irish Economy Thrived (investopedia.com)

SAMHSA. (2016). *Disaster technical assistance center supplemental research bulletin: Challenges and considerations in disaster research.* Retrieved November 27, 2023, from https://www.samhsa.gov/sites/default/files/dtac/supplemental-research-bulletin-jan-2016.pdf

SAMHSA. (2023). *Strategic plan: Fiscal year 2023–2026* (Publication No. PEP23-06-00-002 MD). https://www.samhsa.gov/homeless-housing-resource-center

UN Sustainable Development Group. (2016). *Applying foresight and alternative futures to the United Nations development assistance framework.* Retrieved November 29, 2023, from https://unsdg.un.org/resources/applying-foresight-and-alternative-futures-united-nations-development-assistance

UNDRR. (2023). *Implementing the Sendai Framework, United Nations office for disaster risk reduction.* https://www.preventionweb.net/files/44983_sendaiframeworkchart.pdf. Retrieved November 27, 2023, from https://www.undrr.org/implementing-sendai-framework/what-sendai-framework

Vancouver Coastal Health. (2023). *Supervised consumption & overdose prevention sites.* Retrieved November 30, 2023, from https://www.vch.ca/en/service/supervised-consumption-overdose-prevention-sites

WHO (Ed.). (1998). *The rapid assessment and response guide on injecting drug use.* World Health Organization – Substance Abuse Department. https://cdn.who.int/media/docs/default-source/substance-use/idurarguideenglish.pdf

World Health Organization. (2022). *Foresight approaches in global public health: A practical guide for WHO staff.* World Health Organization. https://iris.who.int/handle/10665/359114. License: CC BY-NC-SA 3.0 IGO

Chapter 7
Mortality, Overdose, and Drug-Related Deaths: How Do We Address Overdose Deaths and Underlying Risk and Protective Factors?

Setting the Scene

> *My older brother Justin Dale Thomas passed away while he was living in a housing unit between May fifth and July 20th, 2023, likely from an overdose... He started engaging in "Illegal activities" at the age of 13, I was 8 years old at the time. ......In my last conversation with Justin, he conveyed regret for the decisions he made during his early years, and he made it clear that many of the challenges he faced can be attributed to that time in his life. He felt trapped in his circumstances, and it is evident that both the justice system and the school system let my brother down. Starting at the age of 13, if he had received the necessary support and guidance, I firmly believe that Justin would still be with us today.......During the last few months of Justin's life, I didn't reach out to him. I was afraid that I wouldn't be able to help him if he asked, and I didn't want to have to say no. I prioritized my own feelings over being there for someone I loved. Now, I realize that what he likely wanted from me most was to simply acknowledge his humanity.*
>
> Tribute from a sister to a brother, Oliva to Justin available at https://www.overdoseday.com/read-tributes/ last accessed January 4, 2024.

Introduction

The story above is just one of many tributes paid by family members and others to loved ones who have died because of a drug overdose. International Overdose Awareness Day (IOAD) is the world's largest yearly campaign to address and end overdose. They aim to also remember, without stigma or shame, those who have passed away and to acknowledge the pain, suffering, and loss of those left behind. The tribute above highlights some of the key risk and protective factors encountered by people who use substances, from a lack of understanding within the school system encountered at an early age, to the sense of helplessness felt by family members. The aim of this chapter is to acknowledge the scale and nature of the challenge,

C. Comiskey, *Addiction Research and Evaluation*, Advances in Mental Health and Addiction, https://doi.org/10.1007/978-3-031-65917-1_7

identify the risk and protective factors and to provide some simple, yet necessary steps to aid prevention, reduce harm, and increase awareness and training.

Scale of the Challenge

The scale of the challenge within the United States was articulated by Nora Volkow the Director of the National Institute of Drug Abuse (NIDA) who highlighted that more than 93,000 people died in the United States in 2020 of an overdose. This was an increase of 30% from the previous year. In Volkow's words, "*The data are telling us that something is wrong. In fact, they are shouting for change*" (Volkow, 2021).

In terms of the global epidemiology, according to the World Drug Report of 2023 (UNODC, 2023d) the number of deaths related to drug use in 2019 were approximately half a million globally. This was a 17.5% increase on the number from 2009. Liver diseases related to hepatitis C accounted for more than half of the number of deaths attributable to drugs. This too has increased in the past decade and hepatitis continues to be a significant global burden. Fortunately, the past decade has seen a decline in deaths attributed to HIV/AIDS among people who use drugs.

Drug overdoses account for a quarter of drug-related deaths. Within these, opioids are the leading cause of death and accounted for almost 70% of the 128,000 people whose fatal overdose was attributed to a drug use disorder in 2019. In some regions of the world this percentage is even higher.

Within North America the opioid crisis is not linked to an increase in the number of people using opioids but rather to the use of fentanyl. Within the United States in 2021 following increasing trends more people are dying each year. Similarly, Canada has also experienced increasing trends in drug overdose deaths and fentanyl was found in 86% of samples tested among those who had passed away. In 2021, Canada experienced almost 8000 deaths attributable to opioids (UNODC, 2023d).

Within the European Union it is estimated that at least 6100 overdose deaths occurred in 2021. These numbers are considered under estimations as many countries do not have up to date data (EMCDDA, 2023a). Numbers within the EU have also risen within the last year.

Within Australia, preliminary figures for what are termed "drug-induced deaths" show that these deaths continue to be a significant public health problem and account for 1% of all deaths nationally registered. There was a minimum of 1788 such deaths in 2021 and this was equivalent to five drug-induced deaths per day among Australians. Records show that factors such as socioeconomic disadvantage, mental health and a lack of access to healthcare and harm reduction services plays a key role in the death of these people (Chrzanowska et al., 2023).

Numbers of drug-related deaths globally are compiled by the UNODC and provided by country within region. Within the Asian region, rates per million vary from unavailable, to a minimum of 0.46 people per million aged between 15 and 64 years of age recorded in 2015 in the Syrian Arab Republic to a maximum of 55.88 per million recorded in 2016 in the Islamic Republic of Iran (UNODC, 2023b). Numbers such as these are difficult to comprehend, however within China alone there were almost 26,000 deaths in 2016. A rate was not provided as there was no total population size available.

Each death within each country was a person and that person most likely had a family, siblings, friends, colleagues. The global scale of the suffering endured by all concerned because of these deaths is incomprehensible. Sadly, the scale of this suffering within Africa is not recorded as data is only noted for two countries (Kenya and the Seychelles) (UNODC, 2023a).

Definitions and Codes

To provide comparable estimates to measure the scale of the phenomena, a common definition must be adopted. As definitions of an overdose, a drug death, a poisoning, or a drug-related death can differ, the European Union Drug Agency (formerly the European Monitoring Centre for Drugs and Drug Addiction) has developed, in collaboration with a range of national experts, an EU-wide indicator to define, measure, and monitor such deaths. The epidemiological indicator has two components, deaths directly caused by illegal drugs (drug-induced deaths) and mortality rates among problem drug users (EMCDDA, 2023b).

Within one EU country drug-induced deaths are defined and recorded under poisoning (also known as an overdose), this includes both alcohol and drug poisoning which are reported separately. These are deaths in the general population due to the toxic effect of a drug or combination of drugs. Mortality rates among people with problem drug use is defined as non-poisoning deaths, which are deaths as a result of trauma, such as hanging, or medical reasons, such as cardiac events, among people who use drugs (HRB, 2019).

As definitions can vary widely, it is important to note the varying definitions used both internationally and locally before comparisons can be made. Within the United States, the Morbidity and Mortality Weekly Report (MMWR) described trends and patterns in drug and synthetic opioid overdoses within the United States from 2013 to 2019. A wide definition was used citing the *International Classification of Diseases, Tenth Revision (ICD-10)* underlying cause-of-death codes X40–44 (unintentional), X60–64 (suicide), X85 (homicide), or Y10–14 (undetermined intent). In addition, drug categories were defined using the multiple cause-of-death codes: synthetic opioids other than methadone (T40.4), psychostimulants with abuse potential (T43.6), cocaine (T40.5), prescription opioids (T40.2 or T40.3), and heroin (T40.1) (Mattson, 2021).

More recently, Friedman and Shover (2023) explored the demographic and other trends in polysubstance fentanyl overdose deaths in the United States from 2010 to 2021 and they also used ICD-10 codes. They selected codes X40-44, X60-64 or Y10-14. From these, they choose overdose deaths with multiple cause of death code T40.4 (synthetic opioids excluding methadone). They then analyzed co-involved substances including methamphetamine (T43.6, psychostimulants with abuse potential), cocaine (T40.5), any stimulant (T43.6 or T40.5), benzodiazepines (T42.4), alcohol (T51), prescription opioids (T40.2-3, other opioids) and methadone (T40.3).

The choice of definition will depend on the specific need for the prevalence estimate and the examples above are simply a sample of what definitions may be appropriate given certain research questions and public health challenges.

Clearly given these varying definitions, caution is required when describing and discussing mortality. When reporting or working with deaths among people who use substances it is important to state a precise definition that can be duplicated. This will enable a common definition to be implemented when comparing across regions, settings, or demographic groups. An appropriate comparison can then be used to identify where an urgent response may be needed.

Biological Explanation

An overdose can occur among people who are new to substance use and who are unaware of how these new chemicals affect their body. They can also be common among people using drugs more regularly and who may require higher amounts to feel the effects of the drugs they are taking. Their body can build up a tolerance and may need a greater amount of a drug to experience the same effect. Overdose may also happen to those who relapse after a period of recovery or those who have been away from their usual daily activities such as people exiting from a custodial or prison sentence, or a hospital stay.

Schiller et al. (2023) provide a detailed explanation of the background and biological and physiological science involved in an overdose leading to unintentional or intentional death. One treatment service provides an accessible description of an overdose for people and families attending their service (Turnbridge, 2021). They explain that an overdose is a biological response to a toxic number of drugs in the body. When too many substances, or too much of a substance, is consumed, it can overwhelm the body and its usual function. As different drugs affect the body in different ways what happens during an overdose depends on the type of drug taken. A summary is provided in Table 7.1.

Naloxone and Recognizing and Responding to an Overdose

The symptoms experienced by an individual during an overdose can vary widely depending on the nature of the drug consumed but it may include some of the following according to MedlinePlus (2024):

- Abnormal pupil size or pupils that don't change size when light is shined into them.

Table 7.1 Effects on the body given varying commonly used substances

Opioids:	Opioids are a class of drugs that derive from, or mimic, natural substances found in the opium poppy plant. Opioids work in the brain to produce a variety of effects, including pain relief
These include prescription painkillers like oxycodone (OxyContin), codeine, tramadol, hydrocodone (Vicodin), and morphine. When they are used in any way other than prescribed they pose a risk of overdose. Fentanyl, carfentanil, nitrazine, and heroin are also opioids that can lead to overdose.	Opioid receptors in the body are activated to slow functioning and control pain. These receptors exist all over the body for example in the brain, the central nervous system, respiratory control centers and other areas. When the body is overwhelmed by opioids these receptors become blocked. The receptors stop performing, and necessary functions such as breathing slow down. The person may go unconscious and stop breathing.
Depressants:	Depressants are sedative drugs generally used to ease anxiety or promote better sleeping patterns.
Depressant drugs come in various categories such as benzodiazepines which include prescription drugs like Xanax and Klonopin. Alcohol is also a depressant. Barbiturates include medications like Numbutal and amytal. These are common sleeping pills. GHB and GBL (gamma hydroxybutyrate and gamma butyrolactone) are also depressants.	Depressants affect the central nervous system. They lower a person's body temperature, blood pressure, heart rate, and breathing. When an overdose occurs, the slowed functioning can lead to respiratory failure, coma, and death. Being under the influence of depressants can also increase the risk of other injuries due to confusion, dizziness or abrupt loss of consciousness.
Stimulants:	Stimulant drugs also affect the central nervous system, but in a different way. Rather than slowing down the functioning of the body, stimulants increase the central nervous system and speed up the messages travelling between the brain and the body
These include prescription medications such as Adderall, Ritalin, and Concerta. Stimulants can also be found as illicit drugs, such as amphetamines and methamphetamines, cocaine and crack.	When an overdose occurs, it can dangerously increase heart rate, body temperature, and blood circulation. This can lead to cardiac arrest, high fevers, seizures, irregular breathing, loss of consciousness, and cardiovascular collapse.

Adapted from Turnbridge (2021) and The Drug Wheel https://adf.org.au/drug-facts/#wheel and The Drugs Wheel: a new model for substance awareness by Adley et al. (2023)

- Agitation.
- Seizures, tremors.
- Delusional or paranoid behavior, hallucinations.
- Difficulty breathing.

- Drowsiness, coma.
- Nausea and vomiting.
- Staggering or unsteady gait (ataxia).
- Sweating or extremely dry, hot skin, blisters, rash.
- Violent or aggressive behavior.
- Death.

According to the United Nations, UN Toolkit on Synthetic Drugs (UN, 2024) an opioid overdose can be recognized by a combination of three key signs known as the "opioid overdose triad." These are:

- Pinpoint pupils.
- Unconsciousness.
- Respiratory depression.

Opioid deaths are primarily caused by a person's breathing slowing down, this is known as respiratory depression and ultimately failure to breath. This leads to the heart rate slowing and eventually stopping, causing cardiac arrest and death. These deaths can be prevented given the prompt administration of naloxone to the person. Naloxone (Narcan) is what is known as an opioid antagonist, and it rapidly reverses the analgesic (pain relieving and slow functioning) effects of the opioid. It attaches to the opioid receptors in the central nervous system and rapidly reverses the respiratory depression induced by heroin and other opioids. It is used worldwide and has no effect on non-opioid overdoses, no dependency potential and it has a high safety rate. The World Health Organization added it to its list of essential medicine in 1983. A nasal spray was approved in 2017 by the European Commission and it has been introduced into several EU countries for use by people who use drugs, their families and services (EMCDDA, 2024).

Five Steps to Assist an Opioid Overdose Victim

The five key steps to assisting an opioid overdose victim include:

1. Call emergency service immediately.
2. Try to rouse the victim.
3. Make sure the victim is breathing.
4. Administer Naloxone.
5. Stay with the victim.

These can be summarized into the ABC response approach as illustrated in Fig. 7.1. Videos providing basic training on this are available (EMCDDA, 2014).

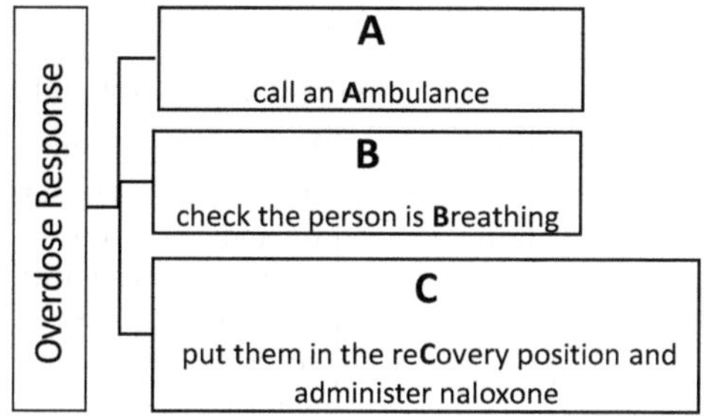

Fig. 7.1 The ABC of responding to an opioid overdose

Stop Overdose Safely

As people who are dependent on opioids are more likely to suffer an overdose a campaign known as, "Stop Overdose Safely," the S-O-S Initiative was jointed developed by the WHO and the UNODC to address this. A Take Home Naloxone (THN) program was introduced in a selection of low- to middle-income countries. These included Kazakhstan, Kyrgyzstan, Tajikistan, and Ukraine. Findings from the implementation of the UNODC–WHO S-O-S training project in these four countries resulted in the reported use of the THN in approximately 90% of witnessed opioid overdoses and noted that the use of THN was especially important in countries where emergency response resources for opioid overdose may be limited (Dietze et al., 2022). Guidelines for others to follow on the community management of opioid overdoses are available from the WHO (WHO, 2014). Walker et al. (2022) provided further analysis of the implementation of the S-O-S initiative and found that in addition to saving lives, participants within the study shared learning, knowledge, and skills. Empowerment, feeling valued and cared for was also expressed by those who used drugs and who received naloxone. However, fear of potential police intervention was also expressed in relation to carrying and administering naloxone.

Preventing Harm and Reducing Overdose Deaths

Prevention of overdose is essential if the tide of increasing opioid deaths globally are to be reversed. The European Drugs Agency (EUDA) formerly the European Monitoring Centre for Drugs and Drug Addiction highlight that prevention will involve a holistic approach, from individuals to communities of practice to policy (EMCDDA, 2023b). This is summarized in Fig. 7.2 which highlights where strong evidence is also available to support these approaches. These areas of strong evidence include the administration of naloxone; the training on, and distribution of naloxone; drug consumption facilities and finally, opioid agonist treatment, retention in treatment and continuity of care.

Within the United States the Director of the National Institute on Drug Abuse (NIDA), Nora Volkow in a blog post in 2022 has also highlighted five areas where

✓✓= Good evidence, ✓= Emerging evidence				
Reducing fatal outcomes if overdose occurs				
Naloxone administration ✓✓	Naloxone distribution and training, specialist services and first responders ✓✓	Drug consumption facilities ✓✓	Fatal overdose prevention apps ✓	
Reducing the risk of overdose occurring				
Opioid agonist treatment, retention and continuity of care ✓✓	Targeted interventions at times of reduced tolerance e.g. after prison release or interrupted treatment ✓	Overdose risk assessment awareness training and harm reduction ✓	Overdose prevention strategies ✓	
Prevention of diversion of medicines ✓	Drug checking and public health alerts ✓	Supporting transition for injecting to smoking opioids ✓	Targeted treatments Naltrexone treatment Heroin assisted treatment ✓	
Reducing vulnerability				
Integrated care with mental health and generic health services ✓	Interventions to improve access to health and social care ✓	Housing programs ✓	Support to employment programs ✓	Interventions to reduce/prevent stigma ✓

Fig. 7.2 A holistic approach to preventing opioid-related deaths and the strength of the evidence. (Adapted from EMCDDA, 2024).

more research is not needed to curb the overdose crisis they are facing. These five areas of established evidence emphasized by Volkow (2023) in Table 7.2 reflect those highlighted by the EMCDDA.

Case Study 7.1: Distributing Naloxone in Ohio State Universities and Schools Within Project Dawn

Introduction

Within the United States of America, Ohio State has one of the highest numbers of overdose deaths registered each year. In 2021 the most deaths ever recorded in the State were registered, with over 5000 fatal overdoses occurring. Similar numbers

Table 7.2 Five interventions to protect people now from the risks of overdosing and where more research is not needed. (Adapted from Volkow (2023)

1. Naloxone Naloxone saves lives, yet despite this it is not available over the counter to ease access and doctors do not always prescribe it
2. Medication for opioid use disorder Medications for opioid use disorder work. Methadone, buprenorphine, naltrexone, and others have repeatedly been proven to work through numerous international studies and clinical trials. Not only do they work but they save money, reduce harm, and improve the lives of people who use drugs, their families and communities. Yet not all treatment centers within the United States offer these medications
3. Contingency management for stimulant use disorders While opioids cause most overdose deaths, Volkow (2021) notes that stimulants like methamphetamine and cocaine are increasingly being found in combination with opioids within people who experience overdose. Even without a Food and Drug Agency approved drug to treat stimulant use disorders, contingency management is an effective behavioral treatment that is available but seldom implemented due to a lack of clarity on its regulations
4. Needles exchange and syringe services reduce harm There is a large body of scientific evidence that demonstrates that needle exchange programs also known as syringe services programs reduce harm particularly in terms of reducing life limiting disease transmission of HIV and hepatitis C among people who inject drugs. These services have the additional benefit of providing an access point into potential treatment options and additional harm reducing measures. Furthermore, they often operate an outreach model and are delivered from mobile clinics which can include service providers on foot carrying a backpack of supplies, on a bike, from a car, a van or a bus. These are known to reach communities where the needs are greatest. An example of a minivan outreach service is provided in Fig. 7.3
5. Proven prevention interventions reduce risks and strengthen protective factors While addressing the current urgent situation with regards to drug overdose globally but particularly within the United States there is a need to implement proven evidence-based prevention programs. Programs which have been evaluated as effective can reduce or delay substance use and increase resilience. They have been shown to be cost effective and avert future costs

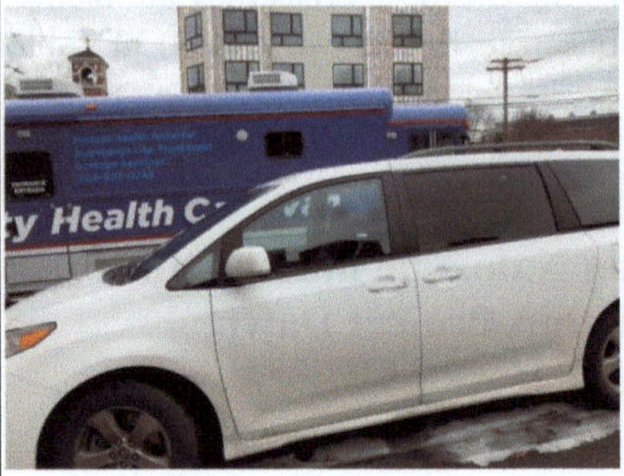

The Yale minivan

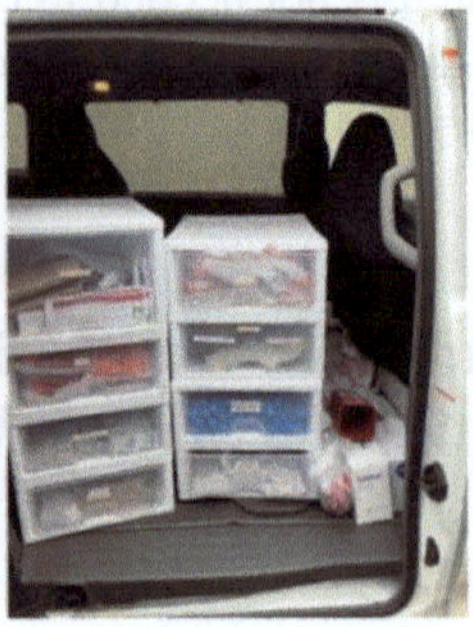

Needle and syringe supplies

Fig. 7.3 Minivan distributing needles and syringe services. (Authors own photographs)

were recorded in 2022 and 2023. Death rates among white residents have begun to fall and this is a continuing trend but death rates among black residents have increased, and this too is a continuing trend seen in the 2023 data. Within Ohio State there are 16 counties, and some have been experiencing increases in deaths while others have experienced decreases (Ohio Overdose Deaths, 2023).

Methods

In response to this devastating challenge for its community the Ohio Department of Health developed Project DAWN (Deaths Avoided With Naloxone). The project works to train community organizations and members to recognize and treat opioid overdoses as well as providing Narcan (a branded name for naloxone) to those who need it including school settings and young people. This project was made possible following the passing of a Senate Bill in 2016. This Bill regulated the distribution of painkillers and pharmacy technician credentials to aid the appropriate sale of opioid medications. Equally importantly, the Bill ensured that naloxone was readily available at schools, homeless shelters, halfway houses, and treatment centers (The Recovery Village Columbus, 2023).

Results

The Ohio State University Wexner Medical Centre partnered with Project DAWN to provide training and free naloxone kits at all of their hospital pharmacy locations (Ohio State University Wexner Medical Centre, 2024). Kits were also available for free for residents by mailing the public health offices directly. No insurance cover was required to receive the kits in the post.

A further novel approach to distributing the kits was via a harm reduction vending machine. This was placed in their recreational and physical activity center and was accessible to both community members and students. The vending machine functioned in a similar manner to other food and drink type vending machines but was free. The machine carried a QR code to enable further information to also be provided. An example of the contents of the harm reduction vending machine is provided in Fig. 7.4.

The machine provided naloxone in the form of a nasal spray. Disposal bags for drug and other related waste were provided. This might include unwanted drugs or expired medications and helped prevent their potential misuse or contamination of the environment. Sharps containers were also available for the safe disposal of needles and other sharp objects related to drug use. Finally, fentanyl test strips were provided to enable people to check their drugs for potential fentanyl contamination and enabling informed decisions and reducing the risk of unintended overdoses (Ohio State University Wexner Medical Centre, 2024).

Within high school settings one district within Ohio initiated training for all staff and yet hoped never to use that training. The school district of West Clermont started storing naloxone in each of its school buildings. This reflected existing policies on storing and training school staff in the use of automated external defibrillators in case of sudden cardiac arrest. The district takes a holistic approach and mandates the education of school goers about drug use prevention and harm reduction. In collaboration with the Ohio School Nurses Association, it was discussed how school goers' access to illicit drugs had changed over the recent past with the use of social media platforms such as Snapchat and how drugs are being disguised and how emojis and particularly emoticons (facial expressions such as smiles or frowns formed by various key board characters) were being used as a language to obtain drugs.

The district's supervising nurse explained that often school goers might think they are getting a drug like Adderall (an amphetamine-type drug used to treat attention deficit hyperactivity disorder, ADHD) to help them study but in fact they may get a far more potent substance containing fentanyl. When the idea of distributing

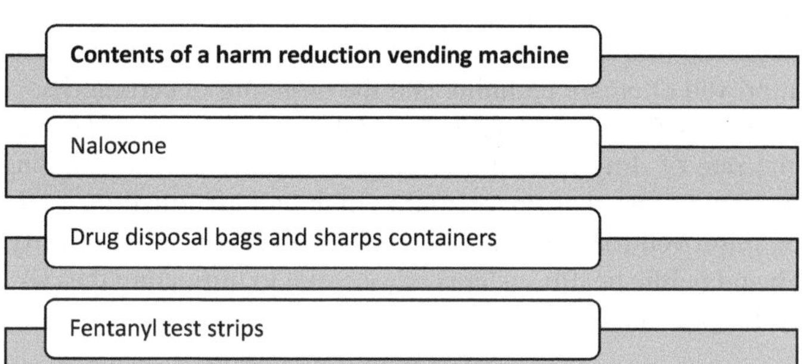

Fig. 7.4 The contents of a harm reduction vending machine at a university location

naloxone to schools was initially presented there was some reluctance among schools however when the program was eventually rolled out no opposition was expressed. All teachers, administrators, and medical staff were trained. Staff know where the naloxone is located within each floor of each building, but school goers do not. The association of nurses felt that the responsibility and decision to administer naloxone in an overdose was too great for students (Mitchell, 2024).

Discussion

These two examples of the use of naloxone in educational settings illustrate how known evidence on the prevention of drug overdose deaths can be implemented using novel approaches. The use of the vending machines for university students, hospital staff, and related community members helps not only in saving potential lives but could also reduce stigma and remove access barriers to this life-saving medication. The distribution of naloxone on each floor of each high school building within a region of the United States that is experiencing the highest levels of unintended drug overdose deaths and ensuring the training of all teaching and related school staff is one further example how existing polices for cardiac arrest training can be adapted and implemented to save young lives.

Case Study 7.2: Reducing Drug Overdose Deaths in Prison and Upon Post-Prison Release

Introduction

The increase in the risk of overdose within prison and in particular immediately following a period of incarceration has been well documented. Zlodre and Fazel (2012) in their review and meta-analysis of mortality among released prisoners, analyzed over 26,000 deaths and found that released prisoners are at increased risk for death following release particularly in the early period following release. They found higher standardized mortality ratios in white, female and younger prisoners. They called for improved aftercare planning and the targeting of certain risk groups.

The World Health Organization Regional Office for Europe (WHO, 2010) recognized that the rate of drug-related mortality, or overdose deaths among prisoners immediately after release was unacceptably high and identified the main areas that needed to be improved to decrease this risk. They identified the priority of linking prison health and public health systems as essential to mitigating the risk and identified the need for preventative responses across all levels of the justice system.

The European Drugs Agency recognizes that people in prison often have complex health needs including drug-related problems, but they stress some guiding principles as outlined in Fig. 7.5.

In terms of equivalence of care, data on harm reduction and treatment interventions available in prisons in 2021 showed that continuity of opioid agonist treatment was available in all EU Member States, apart from Slovakia, as well as in Türkiye and Norway. However, unfortunately initiation of agonist treatment in prison was not allowed in six EU countries. Needle and syringe programs were available in prisons in three countries and take-home naloxone was available in four countries (EMCDDA, 2023a).

The United Kingdom produced a specific toolkit for prisons in relation to the emergence of new or novel psychoactive substances (NPS) also known as "legal highs" in prisons and related overdose implications (Public Health England, 2017). This toolkit covered topics on prevalence, categories of NPS and importantly the management of NPS in prisons. NPS have been defined by the United Nations Office on Drugs and Crime (UNODC) as "substances of abuse, either in a pure form or a preparation, that are not controlled by international drug conventions, but which may pose a public health threat," hence their alternative name of "legal highs." Within Ireland the Irish Prison Service also produced an information booklet on NPS for prison and other relevant staff (Irish Prison Service, 2017). This publication covered details on cannabinoids, ketamine, GHB/GBL, mephedrone, ecstasy, and

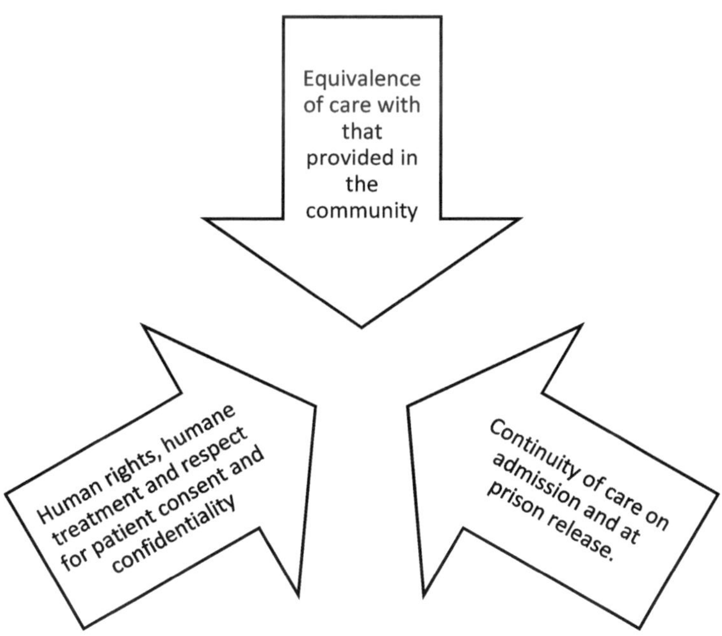

Fig. 7.5 Guiding principles for the provision of healthcare in prisons

other substances. Information sources on the management of NPS in prisons were also provided.

Methods

One Irish prison embarked on the comprehensive training of staff and prison peers to reduce the risks of overdose.

Results

An example of one such training session is provided in Fig. 7.6. The training also involved a live demonstration on how to respond to an NPS overdose. This was recorded and used as training material.

The training was ongoing over a period. It addressed various other substances and varying critical time periods such as temporary release, Christmas time and eventual final release. The Chief Nurse Officer was involved as were peers. The prisoners contributed substantially to the training with peer education in relation to overdose prevention. They actively engaged in initiatives for International Overdose Awareness Day in August each year and a "Staying Alive at Christmas" campaign. Risk of overdose with NPS and other drugs was included in all these campaigns.

Discussion

A comprehensive publication addressing all aspects of the challenges for prison and drugs in Europe is provided (EMCDDA, 2021). Over 850,000 people in Europe are in prison on any 1 day. Interventions available in prison to prevent and control infectious diseases include testing, vaccination, and treatment for infectious diseases such as HBV, HIV, and hepatitis C. Access to testing and treatment remains low. Other harm reduction interventions with proven effectiveness in the community, including needle and syringe programs, condom distribution programs and safe tattooing programs, are available in only a few prisons in Europe and only a limited number of countries provide naloxone to those leaving prison.

According to the EMCDDA, "Providing continuity of care as people move between prison and the community is key to achieving sustainable and effective treatment outcomes, and it is likely to have a significant impact on public health." It is well recognized that the prison and the community intersect as people move between one and the other. While research within the community is well established more evidence is needed on the outcomes of interventions targeting demand as well as supply reduction in prison settings.

SAVE THE DATE

The Irish Prison Service (IPS) will host an information seminar on the topic of

New Psychoactive Substances (NPS)

– the impact on prisons

In the IPS College on Thursday 17th November 2016 from 10.00 to 16.30

The recent increase in the use of novel psychoactive substances in the community is now reflected in a similar increase in use in prisons. This is impacting on the wider prison service and is presenting a significant set of new challenges to prison staff both operational and health care.

It is essential therefore that the IPS considers and plans the approach to the management of NPS, to ensure that staff are equipped to respond to the health and operational impacts of these substances.

The aim of this seminar is to provide information to prison staff (both operational and healthcare) on NPS including the experience in the community to discuss the challenges presented by NPS, in terms of identification screening and treatment and to consider how this issue can be managed within the prison setting.

It is intended there will be a series of presentations by experts in this area from the UK the HSE and IPS staff, as well as a number of workshops to identify the challenges and propose how such challenges can be addressed in the prison setting.

Fig. 7.6 An example of an NPS training day for prison staff

To conclude across the three stages of prison entry, prison stay, and prison release the three principles of human rights, equivalence of care and continuity of service provision should be respected. Further details are provided by EMCDDA 2023c) in their Prison and drugs: health and social responses guide (EMCDDA, 2023c) available at Prisons and drugs: health and social responses | www.emcdda.europa.eu.

Prison settings also produce opportunities for care and service provision. According to the EMCDDA (2023a) they can provide a setting where interventions may reach particular groups of people who use drugs who are often hard to reach by drug and health services in the community. Prisons also support communities, providing harm reduction, counselling, testing and treatment services to people in prison before they are released the well-being of both those in prison and the community to which they return can be improved, producing an overall community benefit. Finally in terms of coercive sanctions by increasing the use of alternatives to imprisonment through a review of the regulations that govern their application and addressing public and professional attitudes to their use may have the potential for improving long-term outcomes and reducing criminal justice spending (EMCDDA, 2023a).

References

Adley, M., Jones, G., & Measham, F. (2023). Jump-starting the conversation about harm reduction: Making sense of drug effects. *Drugs: Education, Prevention and Policy, 30*(4), 347–360.

Chrzanowska, A., Man, N., Akhurst, J., Sutherland, R., Degenhardt, L., & Peacock, A. (2023). *Trends in overdose and other drug-induced deaths in Australia, 2002–2021.*

Dietze, P., Gerra, G., Poznyak, V., Campello, G., Kashino, W., Dzhonbekov, D., Kiriazova, T., Nikitin, D., Terlikbayeva, A., & Krupchanka, D. (2022). An observational prospective cohort study of naloxone use at witnessed overdoses, Kazakhstan, Kyrgyzstan, Tajikistan, Ukraine. *Bulletin of the World Health Organization, 100*(3), 187.

EMCDDA. (2014). *Video: Take-home naloxone programmes in Europe–Overdose prevention.* Retrieved January 23, 2024 from https://www.emcdda.europa.eu/media-library/video-take-home-naloxone-programmes-europe-%E2%80%94-overdose-prevention_en

EMCDDA. (2021). *European drug report 2021: Trends and developments.* https://www.emcdda.europa.eu/publications/edr/trends-developments/2021_en

EMCDDA. (2023a). *European drug report 2023: Trends and developments* ISBN:978-92-9497-865-3. https://www.emcdda.europa.eu/publications/european-drug-report/2023_en

EMCDDA. (2023b). *The future of drug monitoring in Europe until 2030: A report summarising the findings and lessons learnt from the EMCDDA's 'futures study'.* Retrieved December 1, 2023, from https://www.emcdda.europa.eu/publications/technical-reports/future-drug-monitoring-europe-until-2030_en

EMCDDA. (2023c). *Prisons and drugs: health and social responses.* EMCDDA. Retrieved February 9, 2024 from https://www.emcdda.europa.eu/publications/mini-guides/prisons-and-drugs-health-and-social-responses_en#section1

EMCDDA. (2024). *Take-home naloxone.* European Monitoring Centre for Drugs and Drug Addiction. Retrieved January 23, 2024 from https://www.emcdda.europa.eu/publications/topic-overviews/take-home-naloxone_en

Friedman, J., & Shover, C. L. (2023). Charting the fourth wave: Geographic, temporal, race/ethnicity and demographic trends in polysubstance fentanyl overdose deaths in the United States, 2010–2021. *Addiction, 118*(12), 2477–2485.

HRB. (2019). *National drug related deaths index 2008 to 2017 data.* Health Research Board. Retrieved January 4, 2024 from http://www.drugsandalcohol.ie/31275

Irish Prison Service. (2017). *Novel (New) Psychoactive Substances (NPS) information for Irish prison service staff.* https://www.irishprisons.ie/wp-content/uploads/documents_pdf/Novel-New-Psychoactive-Substances-NPS.pdf

Mattson, C. L. (2021). *Trends and geographic patterns in drug and synthetic opioid overdose deaths—United States, 2013–2019.* MMWR. Morbidity and mortality weekly report, 70.

MedlinePlus. (2024). *Drug use first aid.* National Library of Medicine (US); [updated 2022 April 16]. Retrieved January 19, 2024 from https://medlineplus.gov/ency/article/000016.htm

Mitchell, M. (2024). *'It was time': A school district in Clermont County keeps naloxone in case kids overdose.* Retrieved February 9, 2024 from https://eu.cincinnati.com/story/news/education/2023/12/17/west-clermont-naloxone-overdoses/71803089007/

Ohio Overdose Deaths. (2023). https://www.harmreductionohio.org/ohio-overdose-deaths-continue-at-high-pace-in-2023/#:~:text=A%20total%20of%202%2C265%20overdose,died%20from%20accidental%20drug%20overdoses. Retrieved February 9, 2024 from

Ohio State University Wexner Medical Centre. (2024). *Project DAWN and Ohio State naloxone distribution program.* Retrieved February 9, 2024 from https://wexnermedical.osu.edu/mental-behavioral/projectdawn

Public Health England. (2017). *New Psychoactive Substances (NPS) in prisons: A toolkit for prison staff.* Retrieved February 9, 2024 from 9011-phe-nps-toolkit-update-final.pdf. https://assets.publishing.service.gov.uk/media/5a82ee39e5274a2e87dc3b1e/9011-phe-nps-toolkit-update-final.pdf

Schiller, E. Y., Goyal, A., & Mechanic, O. J. (2023). *Opioid overdose*. StatPearls Publishing. http://europepmc.org/abstract/MED/29262202

The Recovery Village Columbus, Schools Stock Narcan in Response to Ohio Opioid Epidemic. (2023). *Schools stock Narcan in response to Ohio Opioid Epidemic*. Retrieved February 9, 2024 from https://www.columbusrecoverycenter.com/drugs/opiate-addiction/schools-stock-narcan-in-response-to-ohio-opioid-epidemic/

Turnbridge. (2021). *What is polysubstance abuse and overdose?* Turnbridge. Retrieved May 24, 2024 from https://www.turnbridge.com/news-events/latest-articles/polysubstance-abuse-overdose/

UN. (2024). *UN Toolkit on synthetic drugs*. Retrieved January 19, 2024 from https://synthetic-drugs.unodc.org/uploads/syntheticdrugs/res/treatment/opioidoverdose/index_html/UNODC_SOS_Poster_updated_November_19.pdf

UNODC. (2023a). *Drug related deaths and mortality rates in Africa*. United Nations office on Drugs and Crime. Retrieved January 10, 2024 from https://dataunodc.un.org/drugs/mortality/africa

UNODC. (2023b). *United Nations office on drugs and crime (2023) drug related deaths and mortality rates in Asia*. Retrieved January 10, 2024 from https://dataunodc.un.org/drugs/mortality/asia

UNODC. (2023d). *United Nations Office on drugs and crime: World drug report 2023*. United Nations. Retrieved August 2, 2023 from https://www.unodc.org/unodc/en/press/releases/2023/June/unodc-world-drug-report-2023-warns-of-converging-crises-as-illicit-drug-markets-continue-to-expand.html?testme

Volkow, N. (2021). *Drug overdose deaths in 2020 were horrifying*. Scientific American, a Division of Springer Nature America, Inc. . Retrieved January 19, 2024 from https://www.scientificamerican.com/article/drug-overdose-deaths-in-2020-were-horrifying/

Volkow, N. (2023). Five areas where 'more research' isn't needed to curb the overdose crisis, National Institutes of Health. Available at: https://nida.nih.gov/about-nida/noras-blog/2022/08/five-areas-where-more-research-isnt-needed-to-curb-overdose-crisis (Accessed: 05 June 2024).

Walker, S., Dietze, P., Poznyak, V., Campello, G., Kashino, W., Dzhonbekov, D., Kiriazova, T., Nikitin, D., Terlikbayeva, A., & Nevendorff, L. (2022). More than saving lives: Qualitative findings of the UNODC/WHO Stop Overdose Safely (SOS) project. *International Journal of Drug Policy, 100*, 103482.

WHO. (2010). *Prevention of acute drug-related mortality in prison populations during the immediate post-release period.* World Health Organization. Regional Office for Europe. https://iris.who.int/bitstream/handle/10665/326483/9789289042048-eng.pdf

WHO. (2014). *Community management of opioid overdose.* World Health Organization. Retrieved January 24, 2024 from. https://iris.who.int/handle/10665/137462

Zlodre, J., & Fazel, S. (2012). All-cause and external mortality in released prisoners: Systematic review and meta-analysis. *American Journal of Public Health, 102*(12), e67–e75.

Chapter 8
Strengths-Based Approaches Addressing Stigma and Trauma: How Do We Address Stigma and Develop Trauma-Informed Approaches?

Setting the Scene

> *My grandfather had an alcohol addiction. Unable to stop drinking, he had taken his own life in a final moment of futility and shame... Overwhelmed by this revelation, I asked my mother, 'Why didn't you tell me until now?' Her response was that she did not want me to lose respect for him or love him less. My mother ... she had seen me speak about addiction as a disease of the brain and not a character defect. Of all people, I was someone she should have been able to speak to openly about why and how her father died. Yet, for her, the stigma of addiction and suicide was more powerful than the scientific understanding I was trying to bring to medicine...* (Volkow, 2024).

Introduction

Dr. Nora Volkow, MD, went on to lead as Director the US's National Institute on Drug Abuse (NIDA) for over 20 years from 2003. Yet we can see from this story that when Nora was 6 years old and living in Mexico City, her maternal grandfather died suddenly and the memory of her mother's reaction still haunts her today. Her grandfather who was labeled an alcoholic had committed suicide out of shame, guilt, and remorse. Nora's mother shut herself away and due to her own shame and perceived stigma never shared the details of her father's death with her children until her dying days. Nora, her daughter, had at that stage dedicated her life to medical science specializing in addiction. Nora the adult, could not comprehend how her mother kept this secret all her life, especially as Nora during her lifetime of scientific work addressed addiction with dignity and respect. The depth of stigma and shame ran deep as can be viewed in this extract of an interview with her.

C. Comiskey, *Addiction Research and Evaluation*, Advances in Mental Health and Addiction, https://doi.org/10.1007/978-3-031-65917-1_8

Historical Stigmatizing Approaches

Lloyd (2010) provides an informative historical account of stigma which suggests a duality of meanings. The word originated from a Greek word meaning tattoo or puncture mark made with a sharp object. This arose from a practice of branding slaves with a pointed stick to ensure universal recognition of their status and to prevent them from absconding. The word has had several meanings including blemishes on the body, such as birthmarks, and marks said to appear spontaneously on people's wrists and feet signifying Jesus Christ's crucifixion wounds. The "stigmata" according to the Encyclopedia Britannica or a stigmatic person may temporarily or permanently have one or more of these wound marks, which may be visible or invisible to others. "*The presence of stigmata is a sign of mystical union with the suffering of Christ, and a genuine stigmatic must have lived a life of heroic virtue*" (Encyclopedia Britannica, 2024).

Unfortunately, in more common parlance the notion of a mark signifying a certain status is the prevailing understanding of stigma. The notion of "*heroic virtue*" while in my opinion is well deserved for people who use substances, is an identity seldom, if ever attributed. However, the association of stigma and stigmatic with suffering is well known but often ignored.

Early work by social scientist Lemert in 1951 spoke of labeling rather than a mark. He described the way in which an individual behaving in a certain way can then be given a negative label by authority figures. This he called primary deviance. If the person accepts this label, it can become part of his or her identity and this Lemert labeled as secondary deviance. This we may recognize as the notion of self-stigmatization in modern day. This deviance was considered by Lemert as being socially constructed and resulting from social interaction between people, with both deviant and authority figures playing key roles in its creation (Lemert, 1951).

Lloyd (2010) citing sociologists Goffman, describes how stigma arises when a person possesses an attribute that makes him/her different from others "and of a less desirable kind—in the extreme, a person who is quite thoroughly bad, or dangerous, or weak. He is thus reduced in our minds from a whole and usual person to a tainted, discounted one. Such an attribute is a stigma" (Goffman & Goffman, 1963, p. 12). The challenge of self-stigmatization is also addressed albeit indirectly by Goffman as can be seen in his comments highlighted by Lloyd (2010, p. 17), "Goffman gives detailed accounts of the manner in which a person's stigma can affect the way in which people respond to that stigmatized person. He also explains how the stigmatized person tends to hold the same beliefs and identity as 'we' do and how the standards he has incorporated from the wider society equip him to be intimately alive to what others see as his failing."

Individual, Institutional, and Structural Stigma

From this historical perspective, we can see that stigma can be found at varying levels of society from the micro level of self-stigmatization to the macro level of public and institutional stigmatization. Similarly, the impacts of stigma can be found at varying levels. Figure 8.1 summarizes this based on Corrigan et al. (2004), who note that structural discrimination can be with or without intent. However, even when intent is not present the consequences in terms of the loss of opportunities and resulting self-stigmatization can be the same.

The consequences of structural stigma can be seen in the numbers globally among people who use drugs who have been denied access to appropriate treatment. Moralizing substance use has had devastating effects on individuals and communities. This has been recognized and reiterated from early treatment provider Jaffe in the 1970s, who said, *"Making something illegal, declaring it to be somewhat immoral, often gets the great majority of people often adhering to that. But it also results in a stigmatization of those who deviate" (*Jaffe, 1971–*3).*

Empowering Language

Fifty years of stigma later, moving towards a positive articulation and inclusivity, recognizing the strengths of people who use substances current National Institute for Drug Abuse (NIDA) director Volkow in 2024, stated,

> *A half century after NIDA was founded, the science of addiction has ushered in an understanding that we can no longer view people who use drugs in oppositional and punitive*

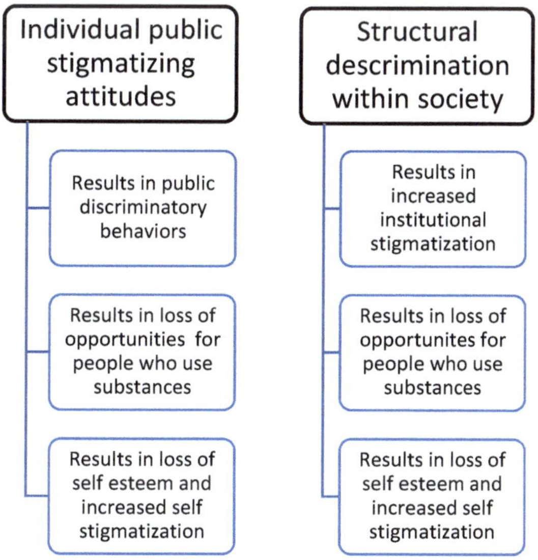

Fig. 8.1 The impact of stigma on a person as a result of both individual and institutional/structural discrimination

terms. The failures of that mindset…have been well documented. People who use drugs can be allies in the scientific search for solutions, and this must be recognized by addiction science. An important component of developing effective solutions must be a community-engaged approach to science that regards people with lived and living experience of drug use and addiction as research partners with valuable expertise (Volkow, 2024).

The International Network of People Who Use Drugs (INPUD) was established through their Vancouver Declaration in April 2006 (NPUD, 2006). This global network aims to promote the human rights and voices of people who use drugs. As part of their work, they have provided a lexicon of positive language to be used when referring to drug use. Table 8.1 provides a summary of appropriate language based on their work of empowering people who use drugs and their communities.

Table 8.1 Positive language choices empowering people who use drugs and their communities. (Adapted from NPUD, 2006)

Language to be used	Language not to be used
People/person who use/s drugs	Drug user; drug abuser; druggo; druggies; drug fiend; acronyms (PWUD, etc.)
People/person who inject drugs	Injector; junkie; smackhead; injecting drug user; meth-head; acronyms (PWID, IDU, etc.)
People/person who smoke drugs	Pothead; chuffer; meth-head
People/person who use/s drugs occasionally or opportunistically	Recreational drug user
People/person with drug dependence	Addict; drug addict; drug abuser; problem[atic] drug user; misuser; substance abuser*; person who is addicted
Drug dependence	Addiction; drug addiction; substance abuse; substance use disorder†
Client/s; service user/s	Patient
Currently using drugs	Relapse; non-abstinent; fallen off the wagon; using again; had a setback; lost cause
People/person who has used drugs	Clean; sober; drug-free; ex user; in recovery; maintaining recovery; ex-alcoholic
Positive/negative drug screen; presence/absence of drug metabolite in screening process	Clean/dirty urine/blood
Communities (of people who use drugs); Networks (of people who use drugs); peer-led networks	Drug using population[s]; affected communities; vulnerable populations
Opioid treatment program; Opioid agonist treatment	Opioid substitution treatment; Opioid replacement therapy

Strengths-Based Approaches

Nigerian author Chimamanda Ngozi Adichie speaking at a TED talk in 2009 spoke of the dangers of just hearing a single story from a country, a community, or a person (Adichie, 2009). When we hear just a single story from a person or a place, we are at risk of a critical misunderstanding. Adichie speaks of her personal experiences when she travelled to study from Nigeria to the United States. She highlights that people's lives and cultures consist of many overlapping stories. When we only hear one story this is often accompanied by power imbalance. In her case her fellow student roommate in America did not understand that Chimamanda had a middle-class upbringing and did not conform to her roommate's African stereotype. Adichie explains that there is an Igbo word that she thinks about when she thinks of power structures. That word is "nkali," which loosely translates to "to be greater than another."

Strengths-based approaches encompass a person's story, their culture and their assets or strengths. Iriss is a Scottish-based charity that works with people, staff, and organizations in social work and social care to help them use knowledge and innovation to make positive changes. Iriss explains that strengths-based practice is a collaborative process between the person supported by services and those supporting them. This allows the two to work collaboratively to determine an outcome that draws on the person's strengths and assets (Pattoni, 2012). What is novel in this approach is that the outcome measurement is a collaborative choice based on the needs and resources of the person rather than on any organizational need or decision.

Macaulay et al. (2023, p. 116) highlight the use of strengths-based approaches in Australian General Practice settings and explain, "*A strengths-based approach focuses on a person's strengths, their protective factors, motivations, and values to help empower the individual and create meaningful goals for change. This contrasts with a deficit approach that focuses on a person's problems or failures.*" These authors argue that by taking a strengths-based approach, GPs can create safe spaces that act as an open door for alcohol and substance use treatment across a person's lifetime.

Four Strengths-Based Approaches to Drug Use Management and Treatment

Ezell et al. (2023) have provided a systematic literature review of strengths-based approaches to drug use management and treatment. They identified and characterized existing paradigms and approaches. Based on their findings they identified four approaches:

1. Harm reduction.
2. Strength-based case management (SBCM).

3. Trauma-informed practice (TIP).
4. Collectivist racial, ethnic, gender, sexual, and intersectional identity-focused interventions.

Importantly they found that these separate bodies of literature demonstrated little connectivity which they then addressed through the development of an integrated strengths-based engagement framework (ISBEF).

With SBCM the philosophy is one of generating client self-efficacy by structuring client engagement around their strengths, skills, resources, and aspirations both inside and importantly, outside of the context of their drug use. The person works towards quality-of-life improvements. Importantly, a key message in SBCM is illustrated in Fig. 8.2.

This systematic review also cited a randomized control trail where SBCM was compared with treatment as usual within an emergency department intervention for people who used opioids. Regis et al. (2020) found that case managers and clients forged a substantial level of agreement in outlined tasks/goals and developed a strong affective bond. They also noted however that although the sample was 75.1% non-white, no analysis of potential racial/ethnic differences analysis was performed. This further illustrates the lack of integration of the four aspects identified by Ezell et al. (2023) Fig. 8.3.

The importance of cultural adaptation is also recognized within the work of the Canadian Aboriginal Aids Network (CAAN, 2021, 2024). Their work emphasizes the need for strengths-based approaches that acknowledge the expertise and knowledge of Indigenous people to navigate complex healthcare systems, as well as the need to move away from the presumption that systems would always fail Indigenous people and consequently lead to poor health outcomes. CANN consists of a diverse team made up of many cultures, gender expressions, and lived experience, all working together within a framework of Indigenous worldviews and traditions. They address HIV/AIDS, HCV, sexually transmitted blood borne infections (STBBI), TB, mental health, aging and related comorbidities and provide a good example of where culture is at the center of their practice (CAAN, 2021, 2024).

Adverse Childhood Experiences

In the seminal work of Felitti et al. (1998) conducted in California between 1995 and 1996, researchers retrospectively measuring the long-term impact of household dysfunction among a sample of almost 10,000 people. These household dysfunctions were labeled as adverse childhood experiences or ACEs. It was shown through the analysis of the findings, that exposure to the traumas of abuse, neglect,

Fig. 8.2 A key message in strengths-based case management

> Measurement of "success" in strengths-based case management is highly personalized.

Cultural congruence (i.e., matching clients with a provider with similar traits) and cultural humility, in terms of attention to multiple axes of identity, particularly race, ethnicity, gender, and sexual orientation, is pivotal.

Fig. 8.3 A second important message in strengths-based case management

discrimination, violence, and other adverse experiences increases a person's lifelong potential for serious health problems and engaging in health-risk behaviors.

Trauma as the result of an event may be understood as, "the effects of experiences that overwhelm a person's capacity to cope. These experiences may be early life events in childhood of abuse, neglect, and witnessing violence, or later live events in adulthood such as sexual assault, partner violence, natural disaster, war, accidents, sudden unexpected loss, forced disconnection from home or culture, etc." (Pompidou Group, 2024).

Adverse childhood experiences (ACEs) have been linked to risky health behaviors, chronic health conditions, low life potential and early death (CDC, 2016). Frampton et al. (2018) found that individuals who had had at least four ACEs were almost six times more likely to drink excessively than were those who reported no ACEs.

The ACEs questionnaire of Felitti et al. (1998) is freely accessible and provides a measure of the number of ACEs a person may have experienced in their childhood and it is provided in Fig. 8.4.

Approximately 60–70% of the general population will experience a traumatic event at some point in their lifetime. Post-traumatic stress disorder (PTSD) and substance use disorders (SUD) are often concurrent. In clinical populations (focusing on either disorder), about 25–50% have a lifetime dual diagnosis of PTSD and SUD. Patients with this dual diagnosis have a more severe clinical profile and are more difficult to treat than patients with solely one of the conditions (Pompidou Group 2018: 5).

As a consequence of the original ACE study, and other subsequent research, healthcare policy makers and providers increasingly recognize that exposure to traumatic events, especially as children, heighten a person's health risks for a long time afterwards. For example, the work of McDonagh et al. (2023) found that the ACE score, the gender and tranquilizer use by a person predicted higher levels of current PTSD among people in treatment for current opioid use. Four of the ACEs experienced during a person's childhood predicted their current PTSD. These four ACEs were, verbal abuse, feeling unloved, living with a person who had a mental illness and living with a household member who had a problem with alcohol or used street drugs. In addition, these authors found that the ACE of, "feeling unloved as a child," was the strongest predictor of current PTSD in adults in treatment.

McDonagh et al. (2023) noted that while summative ACEs predicted higher levels of current PTSD, the factor "feeling unloved" as a child provided the strongest

Prior to your 18th birthday:

1. Did a parent or other adult in the household often or very often…

Swear at you, insult you, put you down, or humiliate you? or

Act in a way that made you afraid that you might be physically hurt?

☐ Yes ☐ No

2. Did a parent or other adult in the household often or very often… Push, grab, slap, or throw something at you? or Ever hit you so hard that you had marks or were injured?

☐ Yes ☐ No

3. Did an adult or person at least 5 years older than you ever…

Touch or fondle you or have you touch their body in a sexual way? or

Attempt or actually have oral or anal intercourse with you?

☐ Yes ☐ No

4. Did you often or very often feel that …

No one in your family loved you or thought you were important or special? or

Your family didn't look out for each other, feel close to each other, or support each other?

☐ Yes ☐ No

5. Did you often or very often feel that …

You didn't have enough to eat, had to wear dirty clothes, and had no one to protect you? or Your parents were too drunk or high to take care of you or take you to the doctor if you needed it?

☐ Yes ☐ No

Fig. 8.4 Adverse childhood experiences (ACEs) questionnaire. (Adapted from Felitti et al., 1998)

6. Was a biological parent ever lost to you through divorced, abandonment, or other reason?

☐ Yes ☐ No

7. Was your mother or stepmother:

Often or very often pushed, grabbed, slapped, or had something thrown at her? or

Sometimes, often, or very often kicked, bitten, hit with a fist, or hit with something hard? or Ever repeatedly hit over at least a few minutes or threatened with a gun or knife?

☐ Yes ☐ No

8. Did you live with anyone who was a problem drinker or alcoholic or who used street drugs?

☐ Yes ☐ No

9. Was a household member depressed or mentally ill? or

Did a household member attempt suicide?

☐ Yes ☐ No

10. Did a household member go to prison?

☐ Yes ☐ No

Fig. 8.4 (continued)

predictor and may represent an overarching risk of post-traumatic stress disorder and continued drug use in later life among adults in opiate agonist treatment. Clearly the impact of trauma is wide and long reaching in a person's life.

Adverse Community Experiences

Adverse community experience has also been recognized as impacting upon health. This is illustrated through the ACEs tree. The "leaves" on the tree represent the symptoms of adverse childhood experiences that can be noticed in clinical, educational, and social service settings, such as a child immunization visit or in preschool or later classroom. The tree, however, is planted in soil that is steeped in structural dysfunction and disadvantage, robbing it of nutrients necessary to support a thriving community. Adverse community environments, such as lack of affordable and safe housing, community violence, racism and discrimination, and limited access to social and economic mobility, create a vicious cycle that undermines the resilience of the tree which represents the community (Fig. 8.5).

Trauma Informed

Trauma is a widespread, harmful, and costly public health problem. It is experienced across different ages, genders, people of varying socioeconomic status, race, ethnicity, and geographies. The definition of trauma can be varied but one is provided by (SAMHSA, 2014) within their manual on trauma. It states (Fig. 8.6):

The manual introduces a concept of trauma and provides a framework for becoming a trauma-informed organization, system, or service sector. SAMHSA identifies the three E's of trauma, these include:

1. The **Event**.
2. The **Experience** of that event.
3. The long-lasting adverse **Effects** of that event.

They then identify the four R's of a trauma-informed approach. These are presented in Fig. 8.7.

Menschner and Maul (2016) have built on the earlier (SAMHSA, 2014) work and developed a brief outlining the key ingredients for the successful implementation of trauma-informed care. They highlight that this implementation involves both organizational and clinical change. These changes have the potential to improve patient engagement, health outcomes, and provider and staff wellness, and decrease unnecessary utilization and wastage of service and person effort and resources. Their key ingredients for a creating a trauma-informed approach to care are provided in Table 8.2. Item 6 within the organization factors is discussed in more detail later in this chapter.

Creating a Safe Environment

Creating a welcoming and safe space for clients and staff is essential (Menschner & Maul, 2016). This involves both the physical and the social and emotional environments. In terms of the physical environment this includes the following:

1. Keeping common areas inside and outside the premises well illuminated with good lighting. This can include parking areas, bathrooms, entrances, and stairwells.

The Pair of ACEs The leaves represent the childhood experiences, the roots represent the community environment	
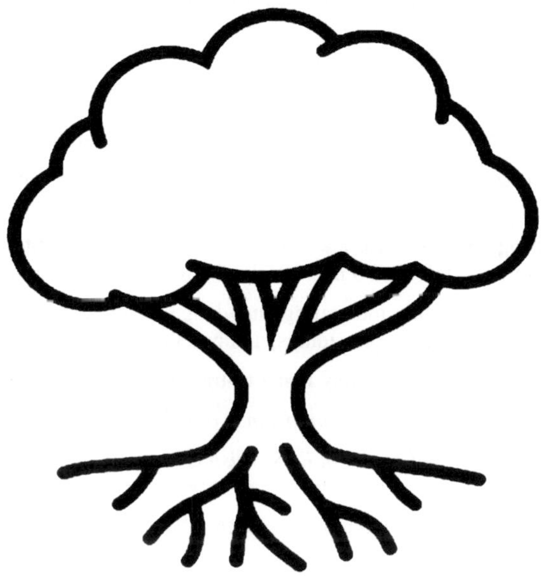	
Adverse Childhood Experiences ACE's	
Maternal depression	Physical and emotional neglect
Emotional and sexual abuse	Mental illness
Substance abuse	Incarceration
Domestic abuse	Homelessness
Adverse Community Environments ACEs	
Poverty	Violence
Discrimination	Poor housing quality and affordability
Community disruption	Lack of economic mobility
Lack of opportunity	Lack of social capital

Fig. 8.5 The pair of aces. (Adapted from Ellis et al. (2022)

> *"Individual trauma results from an event, series of events, or set of circumstances that is experienced by an individual as physically or emotionally harmful or life threatening and that has lasting adverse effects on the individual's functioning and mental, physical, social, emotional, or spiritual well-being."*

Fig. 8.6 Definition of trauma. (Samhsa, 2014)

> A program, organization, or system that is trauma-informed:
>
> **realizes** the widespread impact of trauma and understands potential paths for recovery,
>
> **recognizes** the signs and symptoms of trauma in clients, families, staff, and others involved with the system; and
>
> **responds** by fully integrating knowledge about trauma into policies, procedures, and practices, and
>
> seeks to actively **resist** re-traumatization.
>
> *Recognising the importance of **relationships***
>
> *can be added as a fifth R (Scottish Government, 2023)*

Fig. 8.7 The four R's of a trauma-informed approach. (Adapted from (SAMHSA, 2014) and a subsequent fifth

2. Ensuring that people are not allowed to loiter or congregate outside entrances and exits.
3. Monitoring who is coming in and out of the building.
4. Positioning security personnel inside and outside of the building.
5. Keeping noise levels in waiting rooms low.
6. Using welcoming language on all signage.
7. Making sure patients have clear access to the door in exam rooms and can easily exit if desired.

For the social and emotional environment this includes:

1. Welcoming patients and ensuring that they feel respected and supported.
2. Ensuring staff maintain healthy interpersonal boundaries and can manage conflict appropriately.
3. Keeping consistent schedules and procedures.
4. Offering sufficient notice and preparation when changes are necessary.
5. Maintaining communication that is consistent, open, respectful, and compassionate.
6. Being aware of how an individual's culture affects how they perceive trauma, safety, and privacy.

The importance of the principle of respect is noted in both the physical and emotional/social environments and this is a key value underpinning trauma-informed

Table 8.2 Key factors for creating a trauma-informed approach to care. (Adapted from Menschner & Maul, 2016)

Organizational factors	Clinical factors
1. Leading and communicating about the transformation process. 2. Engaging patients in organizational planning. 3. Training clinical as well as nonclinical staff members. 4. Creating a safe environment. 5. Preventing secondary traumatic stress in staff. 6. Hiring a trauma-informed workforce.	1. Involving patients in the treatment process. 2. Screening for trauma. 3. Training staff in trauma-specific treatment approaches. 4. Engaging referral sources and partnering organizations.

approaches to practice and to care. This value is well articulated by one client who stated:

> *A non-trauma-informed system punishes and blames your adult actions and asks, 'what's wrong with you?' A trauma informed provider will hold you accountable for your adult actions but give you space and time to process 'what happened to you?' without adding guilt and more trauma.*

(Patient at Stephen and Sandra Sheller 11th Street Family Health Services of Drexel University, Philadelphia, PA in, Menschner and Maul (2016, p. 4)).

Vicarious Trauma and Staff Education

It is interesting to note item 6 in the organizational factors for creating a safe environment within Table 8.2. Secondary traumatic stress in staff is not well documented or understood and little research on its prevalence and prevention has been undertaken. Annunziata et al. (2024a) has produced the first estimate of the prevalence of what she calls vicarious trauma among European nurses working in addiction services. In terms of risk and protective factors, Annunziata notes the importance of leadership in this regard.

Menschner and Maul (2016) also note that organizations wishing to implement a trauma-informed approach must provide steady leadership and clear communications strategies to support the transition to trauma-informed care, the engagement of clients in planning and the training and support of all staff including clinical, administrative, technical, and manual workers. They note that building foundational awareness of trauma-informed approaches should begin early in a provider's education and be reinforced through continuing education.

The importance of healthcare education has also been identified by Annunziata et al. (2024b) and she has presented institutional guidelines for healthcare professions (Annunziata et al., 2024a). These are provided in Fig. 8.8.

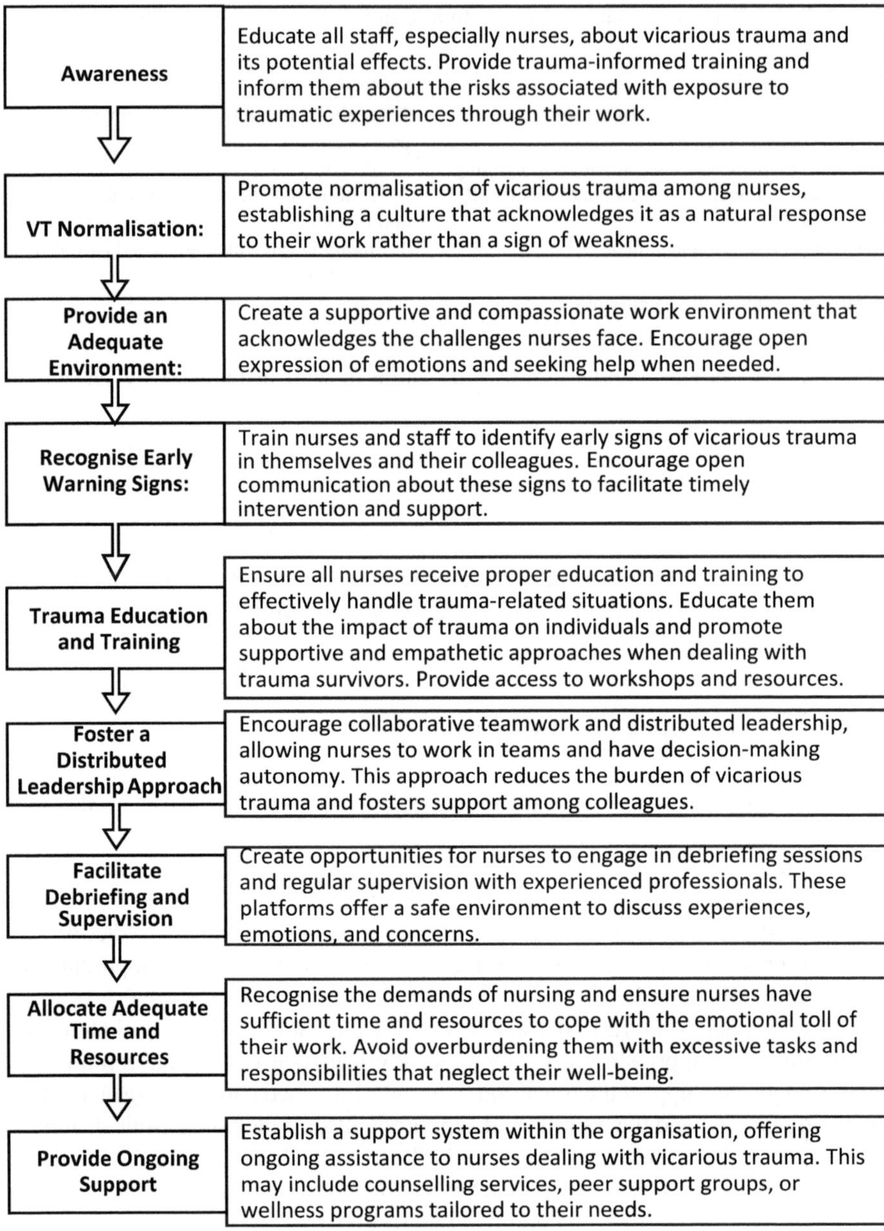

Fig. 8.8 Guidelines for healthcare organization for mitigating vicarious trauma among nurses who work in addiction services. (Annunziata et al., 2024a)

Trauma-Informed Schools

O'Toole (2022) notes that teachers play a significant role in reducing and mitigating negative outcomes by providing strong, stable, and nurturing relationships and creating environments that offer a sense of safety for children. Globally it is recognized that educators need to understand the impact of trauma on development, learning, and behavior. Without this understanding young people's trauma responses can be seen as challenging or disruptive, leading to punitive or confrontational disciplinary procedures and often exclusion from school. This can considerably worsen the overall situation for the child.

Research demonstrates that one of the biggest protective factors during childhood is education. Avery et al. (2021), in a systematic review of trauma-informed approaches in schools found only four programs. These were the Healthy Environments and Response to Trauma in Schools (HEARTS) Model; the Heart of Teaching and Learning (HTL): Compassion, Resiliency, and Academic Success Model; the New Haven Trauma Coalition (NHTC) and the Trust-Based Relational Intervention.

The programs shared core elements of trauma-informed staff training, organization-level changes and practice change, with most program models utilizing student trauma-screening. Generalizability of the findings was weak given the small number of studies included in the review and the variability in the school's studies. Authors noted that further research was urgently required to understand the interaction between core elements of trauma-informed approaches, teachers approach to education and organizational factors that support implementation within schools.

However, in contrast, O'Toole (2022) argues that many trauma-informed approaches within schools lay the burden of change on the individual student rather than on the root cause. She proposes exploring power relations as an approach for understanding emotional and psychological distress and troubled or troubling behavior which themselves can be based primarily on issues of power and inequality. By also drawing on the anti-oppression educational theory, O'Toole argues that a trauma-informed praxis guided and informed by these concepts can help redress many of the criticisms of existing approaches in schools.

To conclude, the impacts of trauma are wide reaching, long-term and costly to the individual and to healthcare providers and those who pay, be they governments, insurers, or others. Together policy makers, practitioners, clients, and their communities can contribute to reducing this burden and improving lives by introducing appropriate preventative early education and current trauma-informed approaches across services.

The enablers and barriers to support this implementation have been addressed by Huo et al. (2023). These reflected known enablers and barriers within implementation science and included the characteristics of the intervention, particularly the perceived relevance of trauma-informed care to the health setting and target population; influences external to the organization, particularly interagency collaboration or the actions of other agencies and influences within the organization in which implementation occurred, particularly leadership engagement, financial and staffing resources and policy and procedure changes that promoted flexibility. Other factors included flexible and accessible training, service user feedback and the collection and analysis of intervention outcome data. Finally, if resistance to change was present within the organization this was a barrier that had to be addressed.

Examples of initiative addressing both stigma and trauma-informed approaches are provided within the case studies.

Case Study 8.1: Addressing Stigma Through the Co-creation of Training

Introduction

In 2018, a voluntary community-based organization known as CityWide launched a campaign to raise awareness and challenge drug-related stigma and the impact it has on people who use drugs. The campaign was called *Stop the Stigma* (www.stopthestigma.ie). The aim of the campaign was to raise awareness of the stigmatization that people who use drugs experience, change attitudes, and move towards a situation where people with experience of drug use are treated with respect and dignity.

A significant issue which emerged in the development of the campaign, was that people with experience of drug use experienced stigma when accessing public services. This finding concurred with a wealth of national and international research (Barron et al., 2019). The participants within the CityWide funded services felt that their interactions with agencies could be significantly improved by providing training to increase knowledge and understanding of addiction and of the personal, social, and economic situation in which the person with experience of drug use lives.

Five key areas of action were identified as part of the campaign and specific actions set out to address them. Action 2 related to the stigma experienced by people who use drugs when they are engaging with public services. Action 2 Challenge stigma in delivery of services, stated: *"We can engage with health care and frontline staff to develop education and training programmes to challenge the stigma that people who use drugs can experience in public services"* *Stop the Stigma* (www.stopthestigma.ie).

Methods

To address this action, CityWide initially commissioned a study to develop a template for a training program that was to be delivered to staff in the relevant public services and which would involve people with experience of drug use in its eventual delivery. The aim of the training program was to reduce drug-related stigma in public services so that people with lived experience of drug use can receive the services that they require in a fair and equal manner (Barron et al., 2019).

The training template recommended a 1-day training program.

Objectives of the Training Template Were

1. To raise awareness of the nature of drug-related stigma and how it can be manifested in the delivery of services.
2. To raise awareness of how this stigma impacts on people who use drugs and on the effective delivery of services.
3. To identify specific aspects of service delivery that may require change and improvement.
4. To reach agreement on how appropriate changes and improvements can be implemented.
5. To assist staff in putting in place a plan for ongoing monitoring and review.

Areas Covered in the Training Template Were

- An awareness of stigma.
- An awareness of drug-related stigma.
- An awareness of drug-related stigma and its impact on people accessing services.
- An awareness of drug-related stigma and poverty.
- An awareness of drug-related stigma as it interacts with other stigmas, e.g., gender, race, sexuality.
- An awareness of the power of language in stigmatizing people and approaches to changing this.
- An awareness of how services can change to become anti-stigma services.
- A framework in which such changes can be made and monitored.

The training program was subsequently developed using a co-design process by people who use the service (co-design participants) and facilitators, and the pilot training was rolled out to public services providers. Finally, the co-design and pilot rollout of the training program was independently evaluated.

To evaluate the co-design process a concurrent mixed-methods study design was used. A combination of observation techniques, focus group interviews, and quantitative surveys were used within an overall implementation science framework. This framework facilitated the identification of both enablers and barriers to the training roll out process from the perspective of both those undertaking and those delivering the training. The survey measured stigma and was administered to service providers who undertook the training program before and after the training was delivered. The evaluation received ethical approval.

Results

From the observation it was very clear that the co-design procedure was respected. There was clear evidence of a shared understanding, of equal power distribution, the use of tools within the process to ensure all participated and the space was deemed safe and open.

From the focus group findings evidence of enablers included the clarity of reasoning behind decisions and the clarity of purpose of the training in terms of raising awareness and accountability. The existence of trust and a safe space was highlighted and the subsequent feeling of empowerment. There was clear evidence of key enablers of stakeholder consultation, leadership, resourcing, staff capacity, organizational support and culture and communication. Barriers to the co-design process were sometimes external practical barriers because of COVID-19 or the need for childcare. Internal barriers were also present from emotional fragility to the perceived scale of the task at hand given the comprehensive and detailed training template (Comiskey et al., 2021b).

The objective measurement of the impact of the training on a small pilot group of 11 public service employees was encouraging. Statistically significant reductions in three stigma measures were found when comparing pre- and post-measures. These three were blame, avoidance, and segregation. A general improvement was noted in all the levels of stigma after the training. In addition, participant expectations of the training were met. These were improving their general knowledge, having better awareness of stigma and self-stigmas, and understanding the impact it has on service users and service provision (Comiskey et al., 2021a).

Discussion

In terms of improving the training, participants expressed an interest in more videos and role playing as this aspect was very useful. In terms of other improvements, participants requested some further clarity on certain materials particularly the theories presented and perhaps more clarity on the breakout sessions that were included as part of the training. In summary, to conclude, it was clear that the co-design process was adhered to with fidelity despite both unforeseen external challenges which included the COVID-19 pandemic. The rollout of the pilot training found that the training package not only met the expectations of the participants but also had a short-term impact on levels of stigma. However as with all community projects the challenges of sustaining the rollout were highlighted given resources.

Case Study 8.2: A Trauma-Informed Approach to Care for Women Living with HIV

Introduction

It has been recognized that historically substance use treatment has developed in response to the needs of men who use substances. Covington (2008, online 2011) notes that counselors focused on the problem of addiction and that other related issues were not addressed. Covington (2008, online 2011) rightly notes that for women, substance use cannot be addressed unless the many related issues are also addressed within services. These include past traumas, current abuse, and additional family responsibilities. She presents principles of gender responsive services which includes relational cultural theory, addiction theory, and trauma theory. SAMHSA (2014) in their practical guide for implementing a trauma-informed approach provide excellent guidance and a ten-point step-by-step approach. They illustrate this approach using several case studies. One of which focuses on the importance of gender and introduces the Helen Diller Medical Center program for women living with HIV at the University of California San Francisco (UCSF).

Methods

The women's HIV program is a trauma-informed service at a primary care center caring for approximately 240 women at any point in time. The director had noticed that while women attending the service were successful in suppressing their viral load, they still had a poor quality of life following their treatment. A trauma-informed care approach was introduced to not just treat the disease but to treat the patient (Rinker, 2019). While the women attending the center all had HIV in common, they also shared a history of childhood or adulthood physical, sexual, and emotional abuse. The clinic director and the Positive Women's Network sought funding and established a five-component approach to care detailed in Fig. 8.9.

Results

The success of the center can be observed in one case of an older lady who was using crack cocaine on an ongoing basis. She was often in the company of friends and didn't wish to use her HIV medication in their company or for them to see it in her accommodation. The center director recognized that a woman's health was a personal affair and suggested that what they had done for other women was to place the HIV medicine in a different type of container, such as one for vitamin pills. The director asked the lady if that approach would work for her. The lady was delighted

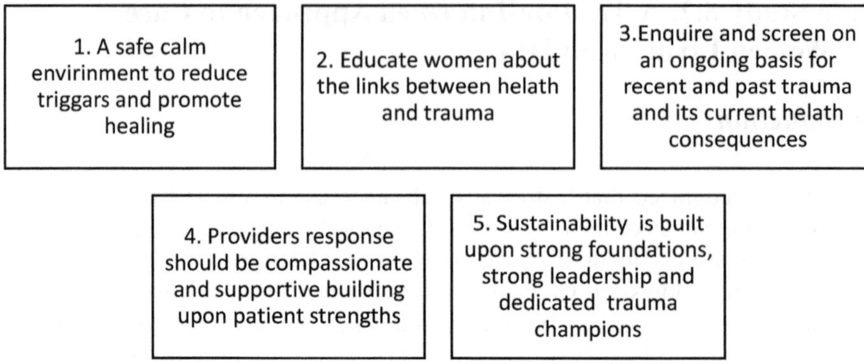

Fig. 8.9 A five component approach to trauma-informed care

and agreed to start her HIV medication with this approach. The director pointed out that for this lady, simply attending the clinic was a success and while her substance use was ongoing she may be able to live and survive in spite of it (Rinker, 2019). This was just one example of how the trauma-informed care philosophy of the center was used to support the people attending and build on their strengths to assist them to make progress in their overall healthcare. This understanding and philosophy can be seen in the quote from the center's director: "*Trauma … the original gateway drug, opening the pathway to depression, anxiety, substance use, health problems, and early death.*" Machtinger, in Rinker (2019, p. 180).

Discussion

From Simone de Beauvoir's seminal feminist work in 1949, "*The Second Sex*," to Caroline Criado-Perez's, 2020 work "*Invisible Women*" the role of women in society has largely been ignored. From early framing of women as other to men in Beauvoir's work to the lack of a gender lens in all aspects of data in the design and execution of product and services in Perez's work. Fine and Sojo (2019) in *The Lancet* special issue on women's health address women's values beyond the business case and while the business and economic impacts of gender is compelling, they recognize that there is a greater need to explore how culture might change when then is greater gender equality. Trauma-informed approaches within addiction polices and services are beginning to take the first steps to address this and build upon both women's and men's strengths while recognizing the ongoing impacts of trauma on health, well-being, and substance use. The latter of which we have learned through countless research, policy, and practice endeavors, cannot be addressed without first responding to the former.

References

Adichie, C. N. (2009). *The danger of a single story*. Retrieved May 24, 2024 from https://www.ted.com/talks/chimamanda_ngozi_adichie_the_danger_of_a_single_story?language=en

Annunziata, K. N., Comiskey, C., & Curtis, E. (2024a). *Exploring vicarious trauma among European nurses in addiction services: prevalence, risk factors, and leadership implications* (in preparation) Trinity College Dublin. Dublin University, . http://www.tara.tcd.ie/handle/2262/147

Annunziata, K. N., Comiskey, C., & Curtis, E. (2024b). A literature review and narrative synthesis of vicarious trauma findings among nurses working in addiction services. *Journal of Addiction Nursing* (resubmitted following minor changes, pending publication).

Avery, J. C., Morris, H., Galvin, E., Misso, M., Savaglio, M., & Skouteris, H. (2021). Systematic review of school-wide trauma-informed approaches. *Journal of child & adolescent trauma, 14*, 381–397.

Barron, M., Galligan, K., & Comiskey, C. (2019). *Template for a training programme on drug-related stigma for delivery to staff in public services*. Retrieved March 29, 2024 from https://www.citywide.ie/assets/files/pdf/2019_research_report_and_template_for_citywide_tcd_anti-stigma_programme_.pdf

CAAN. (2021). *Strengths-based approaches in the HIV, HCV & overdose response, information sheet.* Retrieved March 24, 2024 from https://www.caan.ca/wp-content/uploads/2021/07/Strengths-based-approach-info-sheet-June2021.pdf

CAAN. (2024). *Canadian Communities Alliance*. Canadian Communities Alliance. Retrieved March 26, 2024 from https://www.caan.ca/

CDC. (2016). *Adverse Childhood Experiences (ACEs)*. Centers for Disease Control and Prevention. Retrieved March 26, 2024 from https://www.cdc.gov/violenceprevention/aces/index.html

Comiskey, C., Banka, S., Mcdonagh, D., & Galligan, K. (2021a). *An evaluation of the codesign of a Citywode pilot anti-stigma training program*. Retreiced July 8th from https://www.citywide.ie/assets/files/pdf/citywide_anti-stigma_training_report_final.pdf

Comiskey, C., Snel, A., & Banka, P. (2021b). The second wave: Estimating the hidden asymptomatic prevalence of Covid-19 in Ireland as we plan for imminent immunisation. *HRB Open Research, 4*. https://doi.org/10.12688/HRBOPENRES.13206.2

Corrigan, P. W., Markowitz, F. E., & Watson, A. C. (2004). Structural levels of mental illness stigma and discrimination. *Schizophrenia bulletin, 30*(3), 481–491. https://doi.org/10.1093/oxfordjournals.schbul.a007096

Covington, S. S. (2008, online 2011). Women and addiction: A trauma-informed approach. *Journal of Psychoactive Drugs, 40*(sup5), 377–385. https://doi.org/10.1080/02791072.2008.10400665

Criado-Perez, C. (2020). *Invisible women: Exposing data bias in a world designed for men*. Vintage Publishing.

de Beauvoir, S. (1949). *Le Deuxième Sexe (The second sex)* (Vol. 2 vols). Librairie Gallimard.

Ellis, W., Dietz, W. H., & Chen, K.-L. D. (2022). Community resilience: A dynamic model for Public Health 3.0. *Journal of Public Health Management and Practice, 28*(Supplement 1), S18–S26.

Encyclopedia Britannica. (2024). *Stigmata: Christian mysticism*. Retrieved March 12, 2024 from https://www.britannica.com/topic/stigmata

Ezell, J. M., Pho, M., Jaiswal, J., Ajayi, B. P., Gosnell, N., Kay, E., Eaton, E., & Bluthenthal, R. (2023). A systematic literature review of strengths-based approaches to drug use management and treatment. *Clinical Social Work Journal, 51*(3), 294–305.

Felitti, V. J., Anda, R. F., Nordenberg, D., Williamson, D. F., Spitz, A. M., Edwards, V., & Marks, J. S. (1998). Relationship of childhood abuse and household dysfunction to many of the leading causes of death in adults: The Adverse Childhood Experiences (ACE) Study. *American Journal of Preventive Medicine, 14*(4), 245–258.

Fine, C., & Sojo, V. (2019). Women's value: Beyond the business case for diversity and inclusion. *The Lancet, 393*(10171), 515–516. https://www.thelancet.com/journals/lancet/article/PIIS0140-6736(19)30165-5/fulltext#articleInformation

Frampton, N. M., Poole, J. C., Dobson, K. S., & Pusch, D. (2018). The effects of adult depression on the recollection of adverse childhood experiences. *Child Abuse & Neglect, 86*, 45–54.

Goffman, E., & Goffman, E. (1963). *Stigma: Notes on the management of spoiled identity*. Prentice Hall.

Huo, Y., Couzner, L., Windsor, T., Laver, K., Dissanayaka, N. N., & Cations, M. (2023). Barriers and enablers for the implementation of trauma-informed care in healthcare settings: A systematic review. *Implementation Science Communications, 4*(1), 49. https://doi.org/10.1186/s43058-023-00428-0

Jaffe, J. (1971–3). *Frontline: Interview with Jerome Jaffe response to question: How did the moralizing of the drug issue affect treatment?* Retrieved March 22, 2024 from https://www.pbs.org/wgbh/pages/frontline/shows/drugs/interviews/jaffe.html

Lemert, E. M. (1951). *Social pathology; A systematic approach to the theory of sociopathic behavior*. McGraw Hill.

Lloyd, C. (2010). *Sinning and sinned against: Stigmatisation of problem drug users*. UK Drug Policy Commission. https://www.ukdpc.org.uk/wp-content/uploads/Policy%20report%20-%20Sinning%20and%20sinned%20against_%20the%20stigmatisation%20of%20problem%20drug%20users.pdf

Macaulay, S., Grinzi, P., & Slota-Kan, S. (2023). Engaging patients who use alcohol and other drugs: A practical approach. *Australian Journal of General Practice, 52*(3), 115–121.

McDonagh, D., de Vries, J., & Comiskey, C. (2023). The role of adverse childhood experiences on people in opiate agonist treatment: The importance of feeling unloved. *European Addiction Research, 29*, 313–322.

Menschner, C., & Maul, A. (2016). *Key ingredients for successful trauma-informed care implementation*. Center for Health Care Strategies, Incorporated Trenton. Retrieved March 26, 2024 from https://www.samhsa.gov/sites/default/files/programs_campaigns/childrens_mental_health/atc-whitepaper-040616.pdf

NPUD. (2006). *The Vancouver declaration. Why the world needs an international network of activists who use drugs*. Retrieved March 22, 2024 from https://inpud.net/vancouver-declaration/

O'Toole, C. (2022). When trauma comes to school: Toward a socially just trauma-informed praxis. *International Journal of School Social Work, 6*(2), 4.

Pattoni, I. (2012). *Strengths-based approaches for working with individuals, Iris In-sight 16*. Retrieved March 25, 2024 from https://www.iriss.org.uk/resources/insights/strengths-based-approaches-working-individuals

Pompidou Group. (2018). *Psychosocial support to tackle trauma-related symptoms and related substance use disorders*. Guidance paper, Council of Europe, Strasburg. Retrieved September 6, 2024 from https://rm.coe.int/2018-ppg-3-ptsd-guidance-eng/1680938292

Pompidou Group. (2024). *Pompidou group homepage*. Council of Europe. Retrieved April 1, 2024 from https://www.coe.int/en/web/pompidou

Regis, A., Meyers-Ohki, S. E., Mennenga, S. E., Greco, P. P., Glisker, R., Kolaric, R., McCormack, R. P., Rapp, R. C., & Bogenschutz, M. P. (2020). Implementation of strength-based case management for opioid-dependent patients presenting in medical emergency departments: Rationale and study design of a randomized trial. *Trials, 21*, 1–14.

Rinker, B. (2019). For women living with HIV, a trauma-informed approach to care. *Health Affairs, 38*(2), 178–183. https://www.healthaffairs.org/doi/pdf/10.1377/hlthaff.2018.05498

SAMHSA. (2014). *Concept of trauma and guidance for a trauma-informed Ap-proach SAMHSA's trauma and justice strategic initiative*. Retrieved March 26, 2024 from http://store.samhsa.gov/product/SAMHSA-s-Concept-of-Trauma-and-Guidance-for-a-Trauma-Informed-Approach/SMA14-4884

Volkow, N. (2024, March 12). *To end the drug crisis, bring addiction out of the shadows*. https://archives.nida.nih.gov/news-events/noras-blog/2021/11/to-end-drug-crisis-bring-addiction-out-shadows

Chapter 9
Policy and Practice Development: How Do We Develop a Shared Strategy?

Setting the Scene

Interview with Jerome Jaffe the so called "Drug Czar." Clinical professor and founding head of the first United States Special Action Office for Drug Abuse Prevention during the Richard M. Nixon presidential administration.

> Interviewer: What were the recommendations of your first [1970] report to President Nixon?
>
> *JJ: .... Here were lots of interacting pieces: law enforcement, epidemics and drug use, treatment, and prevention; the government ought to think them through and see how each one affects the other. They needed a clear-cut national strategy.*
>
> Interviewer: What was unique about the approach to the drug problem during that period in history?
>
> *JJ: .... We knew that what we were doing was probably the right thing to do--that treatment helped people, so it was a good thing to make available. But we did not have the data that we now have to show that not only is it helpful, but it's cost effective. In terms of what society gets for every dollar invested, it's terrific. We have that data now.* (Interview with Jerome Jaffe, Frontline, 2000 https://www.pbs.org/wgbh/pages/frontline/shows/drugs/interviews/jaffe.html

Introduction

Jerome Jaffe (1933–present) was appointed as Chief of President Nixon's drug programs in a newly established Special Action Office of Drug Abuse Prevention. He promoted progressive policies and evidence-based treatment, expanding methadone services and recognizing that a range of treatment options from detoxification to methadone maintenance to therapeutic communities were required. It can be seen from the sentiments expressed in his quotes that appropriate philosophy and policy

C. Comiskey, *Addiction Research and Evaluation*, Advances in Mental Health and Addiction, https://doi.org/10.1007/978-3-031-65917-1_9

for treatment was crucial in the prevention of large-scale suffering and the resulting costs to the economy and society.

Globally today, philosophies range from coercive community and institutional detoxification (Yang & Giummarra, 2021) to human rights-based approaches seamlessly moving with the individual from community to prison and back to community (ECHR, 2016). Prior to the development of any policy or practice it is important to recognize and consider the prevailing philosophy. Often this is not objectively stated but rather it can be inferred or implied from popular media sources, government publications, criminal sanctions, and the treatment options that are made readily available. A summary of these philosophies is provided below.

Prevailing Philosophies of Substance Use Treatment

Philosophies can range from detoxification to abstinence-based philosophies, to harm reduction to recovery. Different theories underpin these varying approaches. The Treatment Improvement protocol (TIP) 45 from the Substance Abuse and Mental Health Services Administration (SAMHSA) of the United States Department of Health and Human Services provides a definition of detoxification and guidance on its use. It clearly states that detoxification is not treatment but rather a pathway into treatment and a successful detoxification should lead to treatment entry. They define detoxification within Tip 45 by using the former definition of the Washington Circle Group (WCG), a body of experts organized to improve the quality and effectiveness of substance abuse prevention and treatment. This group defined detoxification as,

> *a medical intervention that manages an individual safely through the process of acute withdrawal.*

The WCG makes an important point when they noted that,

> *a detoxification program is not designed to resolve the longstanding psychological, social, and behavioral problems associated with alcohol and drug abuse.* (McCorry et al., 2000, p. 9)

Often, following on from a detoxification approach to treatment is an abstinence-based philosophy of service provision. The American Society of Addiction Medicine (ASAM) defines abstinence as,

> *Intentional and consistent restraint from the pathological pursuit of reward and/or relief that involves the use of substances and other behaviours.* (ASAM, 2013, p. 1)

Prevention and treatment policies and practices based on this philosophy will reflect this. Similarly, ASAM defines harm reduction as:

> *A treatment and prevention approach that encompasses individual and public health needs, aiming to decrease the health and socio-economic costs and consequences of addiction-related problems, especially medical complications and transmission of infectious diseases, without necessarily requiring abstinence. (*ASAM, 2013, *p. 3)*

A range of outreach and other activities and treatment practices may be included in a policy or a practice with a harm reduction philosophy. Finally, a recovery philosophy can be associated with ongoing and continued abstinence, or it can be defined within a wider context. The ASAM definition reflects this, where recovery is defined as:

> *A process of sustained action that addresses the biological, psychological, social and spiritual disturbances inherent in addiction. Recovery aims to improve the quality of life by seeking balance and healing in all aspects of health and wellness, while addressing an individual's consistent pursuit of abstinence, impairment in behavioral control, dealing with cravings, recognizing problems in one's behaviors and interpersonal relationships, and dealing more effectively with emotional responses.* (ASAM, 2013, p. 2)

Given the ambiguity or perhaps varying of emphasis between the abstinence goal of recovery and the well-being and lifestyle goals of recovery, when speaking of a recovery philosophy it is important to ensure that a common and shared understanding of the philosophy is established.

Theories of Addiction

Theories of addiction exploring why some people use substances and why some people do not, are discussed by Comiskey (2020). In summary these theories can be split into those that focus on populations and systems and those that focus on the individual. At the population level these theories suggest that social networks and the environment and economy are important factors in why some people use or cease to use substances. Policies and practices that support these theories will reflect and target populations and systems.

Theories focusing on the individual may be further sub-divided into two overarching categories. Those theories that focus on automatic processes within an individual and which do not involve any self-reflection for an individual. These theories can be tested in animals. The alternative categories are those theories that focus on choice and decision-making. This decision-making may be rational, involving reason and analysis, or biased, as the decision can be biased or distorted. Policies and practices that support these theories will be focused on the person or individual level and their ability to make choices that are good for them within their personal life setting.

Cutting across the automatic–reflective distinction there can also be integrative theories that combine elements of both, theories that focus on change processes and biological theories that describe the neural mechanisms believed to be involved in addiction.

In summary a range of both population/system level and individual/personal level theories will be present within policies although they may not necessarily be stated. A range of prevailing philosophies may also be present although one may be more dominant than another. Furthermore, these underlying theories and philosophies may not be overtly articulated but rather implied. It is universally expected that prevailing philosophies and theories reflected within international and national policies and practices will be pragmatic and rational as noted by Jaffee (2000). A brief review of the international instruments governing these approaches is provided below.

International Human Rights Instruments of the United Nations

While it is expected that countries will adhere to a pragmatic and rational approach, we will see within the international instruments that where this is not always the case, grave and irreversible harm can be caused.

The founding documents for international human rights are the Charter for the United Nations produced in 1945 and the subsequent Universal Declaration on Human Rights originally produced in 1948. Today the definitions and detailed descriptions of these rights are provided within the Declaration which consists of nine core international human rights treaties and nine optional protocols. The treaties and their optional protocols are ratified or acceded to by States on a voluntary basis. Once a State becomes a party to a treaty or a protocol, it takes on the legal obligation to implement its provisions and to report periodically. There are currently 193 member states. A list is available here (https://www.un.org/en/about-us/member-states).

The 30 Articles of the original declaration in 1948 clearly set forth the broad human rights. In relation to providing and receiving appropriate interventions to achieve one's full well-being regardless of whether one uses substances Articles 3, 5, and 25 are particularly pertinent and are reproduced in Fig. 9.1.

Similarly, the UN Convention on the Rights of Persons with Disabilities (UN, 1966) which adopts a broad categorization of persons with disabilities, reaffirms that all persons with any type of disability, including those who may have a psychiatric condition such as substance use disorder, must enjoy the full range of human rights and fundamental freedoms as an individual.

The Convention on the Elimination of All Forms of Discrimination Against Women (UN, 1979) re-affirms women's rights to non-discrimination in education, employment, and economic and social activities, and protects them against stigma and other forms of discrimination.

The previous international Covenant on Economic, Social and Cultural Rights (UN, 1966) provided further protection and recognized the right of both adults and children to the enjoyment of the highest attainable standard of physical and mental health.

In terms of children's rights, in September 2019, the General Assembly of the United Nations marked the thirtieth anniversary of the adoption of the UN Convention on the Rights of the Child (UN, 1989).

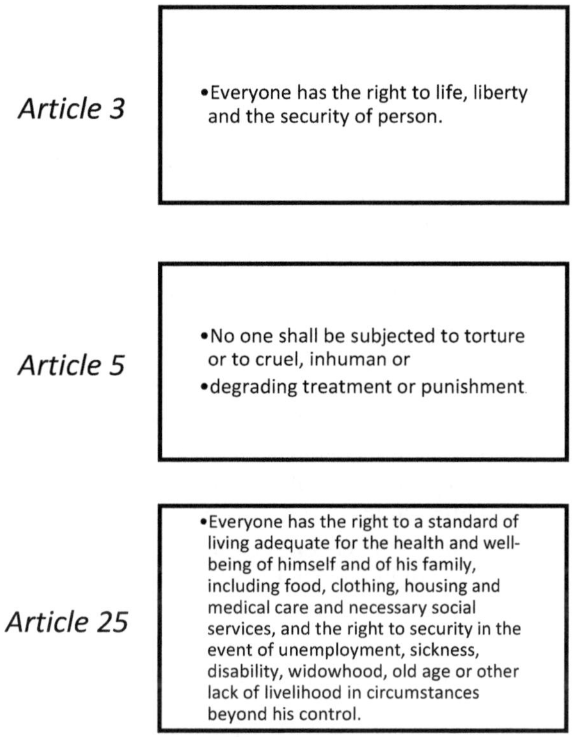

Fig. 9.1 Articles 3, 5, and 25 of the UN Declaration of Human Rights (1948). These Articles are particularly pertinent to remember in relation to people who use substances

> *This is an international treaty that recognizes the human rights of children. It establishes in international law that States must ensure that all children, without discrimination: benefit from special protection measures and assistance; have access to services such as education and healthcare; can develop their personalities, abilities and talents to the fullest potential; grow up in an environment of happiness, love and understanding; and are informed about and participate in, achieving their rights in an accessible and active manner. (Comiskey, 2022, p. 3)*

In April 2016, the United Nations General Assembly had a special session on drugs called UNGASS 2016. The outcome of that meeting was a document which called on member states to adopt proportionate and effective policies and responses to drug problems within their countries. It was hoped that a statement rejecting the death penalty could be agreed by all 193 members including the 33 countries who continue to believe that the criminal justice system is the most appropriate approach for responding to the drugs problem and that the death penalty is an appropriate policy tool. A compromise was agreed and the word "proportionate" was adopted. Within the outcome document the reiteration of the commitment to human rights and fundamental freedoms and the inherent dignity of all individuals and the rule of law in the development and implementation of drug policies was stressed (UN Sustainable Development Group, 2016).

Drug Control Policies

In terms of global policies on drug control, in addition to the United Nations declarations on the rights of people, the International Narcotics Control Board (INCB) is an independent monitoring body for the implementation of the United Nations international drug control conventions. These are the 1961 Single Convention on Narcotic Drugs, the 1971 Convention on Psychotropic Substances, and the 1988 Convention against Illicit Traffic in Narcotic Drugs and Psychotropic Substances.

The INCB works in cooperation with Governments, to ensure that adequate supplies of drugs are available for medical and scientific uses and that the diversion of drugs from licit sources to illicit channels does not occur. In terms of the illicit manufacture and trafficking, the INCB identifies weaknesses in national and international control systems and works with countries to address these. It is also responsible for assessing chemicals used in the illicit manufacture of drugs, to determine whether they should be placed under international control.

In addition to this work, the INCB also produces an annual report within which they provide estimates of the scale of the challenge of the drug control situation in various parts of the world. Each year they also aim to identify and predict dangerous trends and suggest necessary measures to be taken. Within Chap. 1 of their annual report, they address an emerging challenge they have identified and they provide a global picture of the evidence to support countries in addressing this challenge. Topics have included the use of social media in drug trafficking (INCB, 2023); the analysis of trends to legalize the nonmedical use of cannabis (INCB, 2022); Illicit financial flows related to drug trafficking (INCB, 2021); the use of drugs among older persons (INCB, 2020); and improving substance use prevention for younger people (INCB, 2019).

Diverse Global Policy Approaches

While there exists agreed common instruments to guide policy and practice development across the 193 countries of the United Nations, how the policies may be implemented can vary greatly. The implementation of the UN declarations on rights at a country level, will more likely reflect the prevailing philosophies and theories on addiction even though these may not be overtly stated. The original pragmatism and rationality of Jaffee (2000) which may seem a reasonable approach can be widely interpreted.

For example, Razaghi et al. (2023) provide a historical description over a century of drug policy in Iran. The policy approaches included: nonintervention, regulation, legalization, prohibition, and criminalization. The rationale for regulation and legalization reflected the countries need at that time in the early 1900s to generate income through taxes before oil was discovered. Although Iran joined the United Nations in 1945, Razaghi et al. (2023) argue that following the 1979 revolution policies, Iran experienced social desolations, especially during the Iraq-Iran war and subsequent economic recessions. People who use substances have been highlighted to cover-up deeper social problems and authors argue that substance use policies have largely neglected medical approaches as options reflecting the prevailing political imperatives were favored.

Within China, which has been a member of the United Nations since 1945, Tang et al. (2021) provide an interesting modelling analysis of the effectiveness of various potential intervention strategies on the spread and prevalence of drug use . By modelling the existing approach and providing simulations of related alternative approaches authors concluded that strengthening community detoxification/rehabilitation and controlling for relapse were more efficient than anti-drug propaganda or compulsory isolated detoxification.

Yang and Giummarra (2021) provide a discussion of the Chinese approach to policy and argue that the existing compulsory and voluntary treatment models predominantly operate separately from each other and they lack evidence-based guidelines. Following harm reduction philosophies and population level theories, they propose a drug treatment system that embraces social support, psychosocial interventions, and well-qualified health professionals. They support a localized model that is composed of well-facilitated and evidence-based treatment methods for both compulsory and voluntary treatment for people who use drugs in order to reduce the burden of illicit drug use within China.

The inadequate tackling of deeper social problems within substance use policies even when clear evidence exists is not limited to a few politically isolated or ideologically diverse countries. Within the United Kingdom, Holland et al. (2022) remark upon the lack of policy support within England and Wales for safe injecting facilities (SIFs). This is in spite of the rise in drug-related deaths and the established evidence of SIFs role as part of a comprehensive harm reduction approach. Within Scotland, a pilot project has since been approved (Brooks, 2023).

Within Ireland, a country which has been a member of the United Nations since 1955 there have been ongoing delays in the building of the first safe injecting facility. Interestingly, despite a strongly articulated harm reduction philosophy within drug policy documents, the delay was not from policy makers but from local community members where the facility was to be established. This example highlights the need not only for progressive policy makers but also for an inclusive partnership approach to policy and practice development and implementation. A description of the partnership approach to substance use policy development is provided by Comiskey (2020).

Distributed Leadership

It is widely acknowledged that appropriate and ongoing leadership is essential for successful policy and practice development. However, leadership styles can range from authoritarian to heroic centric to so-called transformative styles. Emerging research within healthcare is advocating for a new approach to leadership, one that is inclusive, diverse in contributions and encompasses the voices, positional knowledge, power, and local contributions of all stakeholders working together to solve challenges. According to Curtis et al. (2021), distributed leadership (DL) has emerged as an innovative alternative to the traditional top-down leadership structure. Distributed leadership enables the action and influence of people at all levels within an organization and supports interventions from wider communities of health professionals.

Beirne (2021) notes that leadership qualities and interventions can be found at all levels of an organization in the interactions of groups of people as they work together to solve local problems. Leadership can be spontaneous as particular individuals' step in and out of leadership activities, voluntarily sharing them with colleagues as the need arises. Local understandings and agreements can be negotiated below the radar of formal hierarchical leadership structures and can even compensate when the formal leadership is lacking.

O'Neill et al. (2021) highlight this disconnect and the competing values that can often be found when implementing healthcare reform. Comiskey et al. (2021) provides examples of how DL can work to enhance advanced nursing practice by bringing about local change that addresses patient needs.

Distributed leadership does not advocate for the removal of positional authority. Within DL, positional authority is considered to be vital for enabling and supporting DL, for facilitating participative decision-making and for providing opportunities within an organization for ordinary leaders to make a contribution and to be encouraged and recognized for the differences they make.

Partnership Approaches

Partnership, according to the Institute for Capacity Strengthening (2015), is a relationship based on mutual commitment and complementary purpose and values that is often supported by shared resources and which results in positive change and increased social justice. Successful partnerships require a good understanding of the principles that make the relationship strong, demonstrated evidence of respectful attitudes and ongoing focus on strong relationship fostering and management of the partnership during the process of development and attainment of the partnership goals.

An example of agreed partnership principles expressed by a partnership of voluntary, community and statutory sectors in the sharing of health and social care are provided in Fig. 9.2. The establishment of these principles are the fundamental building block of a successful partnership.

An example of these principles in action can be found in the development of a national drug strategy described by Comiskey (2020). This example also discusses the challenges that can arise and how consensus needs to be obtained which can be problematic but also rewarding when a common goal across partners is achieved.

Within the criminal justice setting Marder (2024) provides a further example of how a broad network of partners can be developed with a shared vision, mission, and goals for enhanced criminal justice research for the development of evidence informed policy and practice.

Case Study 9.1: Using Distributed Leadership and a Partnership Approach to Change Nursing Practice: The Healthy Addiction Treatment (HAT) Nursing Model

Introduction

Within busy city addiction treatment centers the workload of nursing staff is often the full caseload of clients registered at the center. Nursing professionals are often practicing in a reactive manner to the daily challenges emerging and presenting among clients. This can lead to fragmented practice with little time for long term planning and care of patients along their treatment journey. Nurses working in addiction services can be faced with a myriad of healthcare conditions from acute and chronic infectious disease management of HIV and Hepatitis C; maintenance of non-communicable disease care from diabetes to hypertension; mental health challenges of acute anxiety to post-traumatic stress and from routine wound care and bandaging to treating lacerations and injuries from falls.

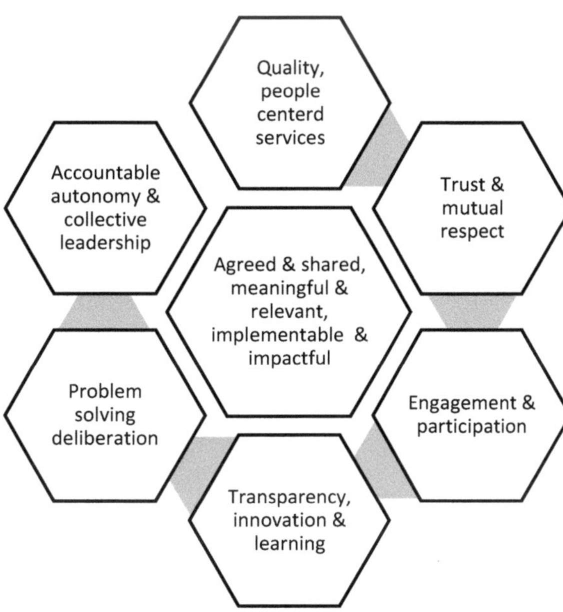

Fig. 9.2 Agreed partnership principles for health and social care sectors working with the state. (Adapted from Health Service Executive, 2023)

Within one city clinic, nursing staff collectively decided to address their model of practice in partnership with their clients and with their local university nursing department. The team identified their core skills as outlined in Table 9.1.

The team's client base involved adults with primarily opiate addiction and poly drug use including alcohol use. Clients exhibited multiple psychosocial complexities detailed in Table 9.2. The nursing teams served their clients across the city in seven drug treatment centers and seven satellite clinics over 7 days a week.

An earlier external review of the existing model for nursing services within these addiction clinics had been described as task oriented and reactive with little time for flexibility in work practice, reflection on client need, or scope for innovation (Strang, 2011). Yet, in a review of conceptual models to guide nursing and midwifery in the community, Leahy-Warren et al. (2017) stated the priority of the focus of nursing should be on client need. Authors noted that a model that depicts a person on a preventative–curative journey within their lifespan is suitable and that the health-related needs of the client, in line with their position in the curative pathway should determine the nurse or midwife intervention.

Methods

The local nursing leadership took a distributed leadership approach to her team and the team recognized that they needed a wider partnership collaboration to identify and address the challenge. The distributed leadership approach was not overtly stated but was evident in how all team members were able to contribute given their

Table 9.1 Core addiction nursing skills

Community health
Addiction
Alcohol management
Drug detoxification
Sexual health
Mental health
Blood-borne viruses
Infection control
Maternity health
Contraception
Criminality
Coaching
Issue viability/wound management
Organizational management
Chronic diseases (example: asthma, diabetes)
Palliative care counselling

Table 9.2 Sample of the psychosocial complexities within an addiction nursing client case load

Psychosocial complexities
Homelessness
Poverty
Early school leavers
Endured adverse childhood events
Involved in criminal activity
Marginalized
Multiple pregnancies
Children not living with their mothers
Children in kinship care or foster care
Dual diagnosis was common
Ageing cohort
Chronic illnesses

local expertise. This expertise may have been obtained within an infectious disease clinic at the local acute hospital, or the maternity clinic run by the midwife working with women who use drugs or within the methadone dispensing clinic. The partnership was expanded beyond the nursing team to clients attending the service and to an academic university-based nursing team who assisted with the study design and execution.

To objectively measure client needs a cross-sectional study was conducted using validated survey Instrument known as the Opiate Treatment Index (OTI; Darke et al. (1991). This instrument includes the 28-item General Health Questionnaire (GHQ-28) (Goldberg, 1978; Sterling, 2011). The OTI consists of a standardized range of measures covering six main outcome domains, which are drug use, HIV risk-taking behavior, social functioning, criminality, health status, and psychological adjustment, as measured by the GHQ-28. This instrument reflected the sample of the psychosocial complexities within an addiction nursing client case load. Descriptive statistics, 95% confidence intervals, and chi-square tests of independence or Fisher exact tests, as appropriate, were prepared for all subscales of the OTI and the GHQ-28. Q scores were also computed for the substance use subscale of the OTI. Details are provided in Comiskey (2021).

To understand the subjective needs of clients, all clients in the study were invited to provide their feedback on the nursing service through a range of open-ended interview questions. Interviews were analyzed using thematic analysis taking an inductive approach.

Finally, to inform the addiction nursing model design findings were supplemented by a mapping of key features from existing established nursing models that were considered relevant by the nursing team and practical to implement in an addiction nursing context.

Results

One hundred thirty-one clients (6.5% of the caseload of approximately 2000 clients) from a representative sample of addiction service clinics specializing in methadone treatment, from a sample frame of 17, were interviewed from May to November 2017. Clients were eligible for inclusion in the study if they were attending any of these methadone satellite or dispensing treatment clinics in the area, were over 18 years old, and were prepared to provide written consent.

In terms of qualitative findings, clients articulated the role of the nurse in their physical care; however, unexpectedly, clients identified nurses as an essential source of psychological support and expressed the wish for the role to be expanded in terms of managing methadone treatment and accessing additional services and resources (Comiskey, 2019).

The quantitative findings demonstrated that the mean age of the clients was 41 years with a range from 26 to 66 years. More than one third (36%) left school before the age of 15 years, 90% were not employed at the time of the interview. Sixty-two percent of the clients lived in a rented accommodation or in their own homes. In addition, 61% had children under the age of 18 years; of these, over half (56%) did not have their children living with them. All clients responding were on a substitution treatment program. The mean methadone dose was 67 ml, and the range was from 0 to 160 ml. On average, clients had spent 7.8 years in their current treatment, and this ranged from 6 weeks to 26 years. This length of duration in current treatment reflected the prevailing harm reduction philosophy. Section 6 of the OTI measured physical health symptoms.

The main finding was how little men and women differed in their experiencing of symptoms, with the most common health symptom across both genders being fatigue and energy loss, which were experienced by over 80% of women and 70% of men in the last month. Section 7 of the OTI measures psychological adjustment. The mean overall score of participants was 8.83 (SD = 7.55) indicating that, on average, participants scored above the recommended cutoff point of 4. In addition, it was observed that 60.7% (n = 52) of all participants had a score of 5 or more. Among women, this rose to 73.4% (n = 22), and among men, 53.6% (n = 29) had a score of 5 or more (Comiskey, 2021).

Given these results on the objective measurement of client need, it was clear that trauma and psychological adjustment was a priority need of clients attending the addiction nursing services.

Following the review of the nursing models by the nursing and midwifery team, consensus arose and it was decided that any model developed must address client needs; hence, it must be adaptable with time, be nurse-led, be measurable and implementable. It must be cognizant of the person and the environment (both the clinic and the community) and it must have a biopsychosocial approach and possibly use a brief intervention approach to target a single measurable behavioral change outcome.

Given the summary of key features, a nurse-led, collaborative approach with a hybrid model was recommended. While a nurse may work with an individual using the FRAMES brief intervention approach for a targeted outcome, the HAT model is targeted at a health and recovery need at the local population level. It could be viewed as a health promotion model. The broad conceptual model that is operationalized in nursing practice is underpinned by a logic model. A logic model is used for illustration; the nurse-led, Healthy Addiction Treatment (HAT) Recovery Model is presented in Fig. 9.3 and a localized operational logic model for the nursing and midwifery team is presented in Table 9.3.

Discussion

From the synthesis of all key findings the Health Addiction Treatment (HAT) recovery nursing model was proposed by the academic team and was ultimately finalized and implemented in partnership with the practice team and their clients (Flanagan, 2022). Results contributed to the formation of the nurse-led, client mental-health-focused, Healthy Addiction Treatment Recovery Model for addiction nursing services.

In terms of national policies, findings provided new evidence articulated by service users on their desire for the expansion of nurse prescribing in addiction services and an expansion of the role to address client needs more adequately. The evidence for the expanded nurse prescribing role was later supported by a systematic review of nurse prescribing practices in addiction by Banka-Cullen et al. (2023).

Case Study 9.2: International Drug Policy Development and the Pompidou Group

Introduction

Many may have seen the original and award winning 1971 film "The French Connection" with Gene Hackman, Roy Scheider, and Fernando Rey. What viewers may not know is that it is based on Robin Moore's 1969 nonfiction book of the same name which tells the story of narcotics detectives in pursuit of a French heroin smuggler. Around the same time that this book was being written Jerome Jaffe was writing his first report on the drug use within the United States. At the same time in 1971 the then French president Georges Pompidou was crafting a letter to the Prime Ministers of Germany, Belgium, Italy, Luxembourg, the Netherlands, and the United Kingdom expressing his concerns amid growing international pressure to control the "French connection" which was a large-scale smuggling route through which heroin was shipped from Turkey to the United States. In his letter, Pompidou says:

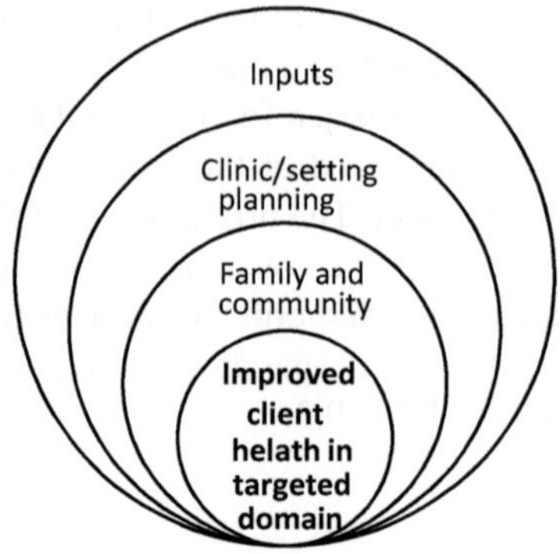

Inputs	Clinic/setting planning	Family and community
• Funding • HAT nursing model manual • Nurse champion • Local area services support: information, training and access	• Development of links with families • Case management team • Development of links between	• Increase access for families to local services • Increased involvement of families and the community in the clinic
• Funders implementation support.	clinic, service and community • Leadership, management and ownership • Staff continuing professional development.	• Increased client knowledge and awareness of health and wellbeing • Enhanced staff knowledge, awareness and skills.

Fig. 9.3 The nurse-led, healthy Addiction Treatment (HAT) recovery model

The dramatic increase in drug addiction is very worrying. While it first appeared to strike the United States, where the president has underlined the need for vigorous action, there is no question that Europe in turn has been affected by this scourge. Young people, in particular, are being attracted by a fashion that is still relatively limited but is leading to increasing use of terrible drugs whose effects are destructive for the personality, when they are not fatal.

(Pompidou, sixth August 1971, letter https://www.coe.int/en/web/pompidou/about/history)

Following this initiative, the intergovernmental body The Co-operation Group to Combat Drug Abuse and Illicit Trafficking in Drugs was formed in 1971. Until 1979, the group operated without a formal status supported by the countries holding its presidency: France from 1971 to 1977 and Sweden from 1977 to 1979. The group developed as a "sui generis" entity (a Latin phrase that translates to "of its own kind") throughout the 1970s. Three other countries, Denmark, Ireland, and Sweden joined it during that decade all working in partnership to address a common mission.

Table 9.3 A localized HAT logic model for addiction nursing practice, with short-, medium-, and longer-term goals

Needs	Activities	Short-term goals	Medium-/ long-term goals
Clients Mental health support need identified by clients in research. Staff Education in SAOR, WRAP, trauma-Informed approach, anxiety, depression, self-esteem, stress, suicidal ideation and self-harm and any other mental health issues as deemed necessary	**Implementation in practice stage 1** 30 clients will be randomly selected from the clients in original sites **Commitment to sessions** Clients to be asked to commit to six sessions **Did not attend (DNA)** If client DNA first appointment, client to be contacted and reason for DNA documented in client nursing records for both pilots. Second appointment to be offered and any further DNA documented with reason why. **Length of session** 45 minutes client interaction, 15 min to document interaction. **Assessment** through Core 10 and SAOR followed by introduction of the HAT Recovery care plan for six sessions. Copy of care plan to be given to client throughout the sessions and care plan can be copied and pasted into care plan interaction under procedures and tests on DAIS (clinic data system) Folders with assessment tools and care plans to be kept in each location and also in the shared folder. Mental health resource information to be available for clients in every location. Clients will either be discharged or referred to other professionals for on-going support following six sessions.	Identification of triggers which will help the client prevent and respond to anxiety, stress low self-esteem, depression, self-harm and suicide ideation Development of safety plan. Completion of 6-week WRAP program. Provision of information on local support services. Clients supported and risks identified with appropriate / timely referral to counselling and mental health services. Symptom reduction. Reduction in external service use (primary care etc.) Reduction in stigma associated with seeking mental health or behavioral health services	Clear pathway for clients presenting with stress, anxiety, low self-esteem depression, self-harm, suicidal. Improved mental health and wellness. Improved quality of life. Reduction in number of crisis interventions. Improved social skills. Improved activities of daily living skills. Improved use of evidence and data. Shared learning re best practice. Improved relationships. Reduce stigma associated with seeking mental health or behavioral health services

The mission of the Pompidou Group is to provide knowledge, support, and solutions for effective, evidence-based drug policies, which fully respect human rights. It is an integral part of the Council of Europe, the institutional guardian of human rights within Europe. The Group upholds the principle that human rights are a transversal issue that are to be considered in all activities to help member states meet their obligations under the Council of Europe and United Nations conventions in the delivery of their drug policies.

In June 2021 on the Group's 50th anniversary, their statues were updated to extend the focus of their work to include addictive behaviors related to licit substances such as alcohol and tobacco and new forms of addiction. They implemented a stronger focus on human rights as they are the only international drug policy platform with a statutory mission to promote and protect the rights of people and they reinformed a multidisciplinary approach to addressing drug challenges. Which they rightly believe can only be tackled effectively if policy, practice, and science are linked.

Methods

Evidence for this multidisciplinary partnership approach to policy and practice can be seen in the Pompidou Groups work. The group introduced a subject they believed had not received sufficient attention, the subject of children of parents who use drugs. Using a cross country and institution partnership approach their work addresses both the children and parents affected by substance use while focusing on the programs, services, and practices in place in the different states to address the issue. The project on children whose parents use drugs has been carried out in two phases: the first one started in November 2020 and was completed in February 2021. The second phase has been implemented throughout 2021 with the involvement of 11 countries (Croatia, Cyprus, Greece, Iceland, Ireland, Italy, Mexico, Poland, Romania, Switzerland, and Turkey).

Results

The finding from this body of work of the Pompidou Group and its partners can be found in a series of four volumes each representing a different aspect of this global challenge. Volume 1 identifies promising practices and recommendations that other policy makers and practitioners can use as a guide for their own development of services. Volume 2, "We are Warriors" discuss the challenges experienced by mothers who use drugs. Volume 3, "Listen to the Silence of the Child," explores the experiences of 33 children from five different countries. Finally volume 4 provides a view on how to develop more comprehensive, child-centered approaches in drug policies in general and in non-stigmatizing drug treatment and care in particular (Pompidou Group, 2024) (Fig. 9.4).

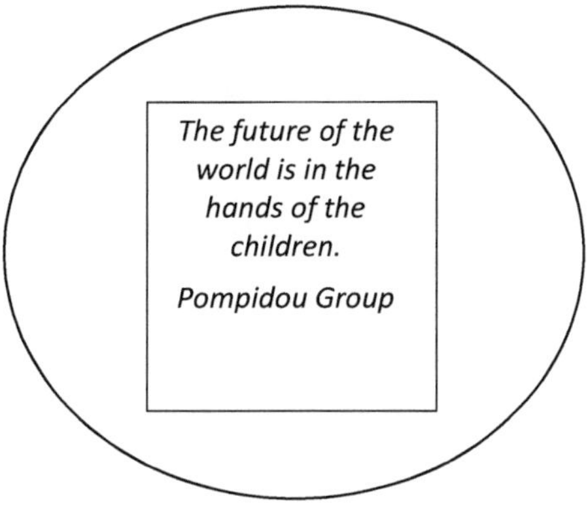

Fig. 9.4 The Pompidou Group's work on children of parental who use drugs, representing the fact that the future world is in their hands Children whose parents use drugs—Pompidou Group (coe.int)

Discussion

This body of work is the outcome of international partnership and collaboration among researchers, practitioners, and policy makers at different levels. It provides essential steps toward the ultimate goal of mainstreaming human rights including children's rights into drug policy. Levels of partnership included country member level, individual contributor level, service provider level, and service user level including mothers, fathers, and children.

This project was originally proposed in response to the Council of Europe's invitation to Pompidou Group Secretariat to contribute to the discussions on the themes which should appear in the new Council of Europe Strategy on the Rights of the Child for the period 2022–2027. Thanks to the involvement and contribution of the Pompidou Group, the Council of Europe Strategy on the Rights of the Child contains the objective *"Mapping, analysing and providing guidance on the situation of children suffering from addictive behaviours and children of parents using drugs."* By this inclusion in the Council of Europe's Strategy, it ensures that this essential topic will receive statutory recognition across Europe and will, it is hoped, lead to the betterment of children everywhere.

In the words of United Nations Secretary-General, António Guterres,

> *In the end, it comes down to values, as was said so many times today. We want the world our children inherit to be defined by the values enshrined in the UN Charter: peace, justice, respect, human rights, tolerance and solidarity. (*UN, 2016*).*

References

ASAM. (2013). *Terminology related to addiction, treatment, and recovery*. American Society of Addiction Medicine. Retrieved February 20, 2024 from https://www.chestnut.org/resources/d4f07c9d-0cc1-44fc-a2a8-5640e60024a2/ASAM-Recovery-Terminology-2013.pdf

Banka-Cullen, S. P., Comiskey, C., Kelly, P., Zeni, M. B., Gutierrez, A., & Menon, U. (2023). Nurse prescribing practices across the globe for medication-assisted treatment of the opioid use disorder (MOUD): A scoping review. *Harm Reduction Journal, 20*(1), 78.

Beirne, M. (2021). Chapter 1. Introducing the collection: A leadership book like no other! In E. Curtis, M. Beirne, J. Cullen, R. Norway, & S. Corrigan (Eds.), *Distributed leadership in nursing and healthcare* (pp. 1–16). Open University Press.

Brooks, L. (2023). *Glasgow gets go-ahead to open UK's first drug consumption room*. Retrieved February 22, 2023 from https://www.theguardian.com/uk-news/2023/sep/27/glasgow-gets-go-ahead-open-uk-first-drug-consumption-room

Comiskey, C. (2019). *Addiction debates: Hot topics from policy to practice*. Sage. https://us.sagepub.com/en-us/nam/addiction-debates/book269028

Comiskey, C. (2020). Reducing harm, supporting recovery: A partnership and evidence-informed approach to developing the new Irish health led, National Drug Strategy. *Harm Reduction Journal, 17*(1), 3.

Comiskey, C. (2021). Chapter 9. Distributed leadership interventions at advanced clinical practitioner level. In E. Curtis, M. Beirne, J. Cullen, R. Norway, & S. Corrigan (Eds.), *Distributed Leadership in Nursing and Healthcare*. Open University Press.

Comiskey,C.M.(2022).*Responsestotheneedsofchildrenofparentswhousedrugs*.EMCDDA.https://www.emcdda.europa.eu/drugs-library/responses-needs-children-people-who-use-drugs_en

Comiskey, C., Galligan, K., Flanagan, J., Deegan, J., Farnann, J., & Hall, A. (2021). The healthy addiction treatment recovery model: Developing a client-driven, nurse-led addiction nursing model. *Journal of Addictions Nursing, 32*(1), E11–E20.

Curtis, E. A., Beirne, M., Cullen, J., Northway, R., & Corrigan, S. (2021). *Distributed leadership in nursing and healthcare: Theory, evidence and development*. McGraw-Hill Education.

Darke, S. et al. (1991) *The opiate treatment index (OTI) manual*. Publication. Available at: https://ndarc.med.unsw.edu.au/sites/default/files/ndarc/resources/TR.011.pdf. Accessed 03 June 2024.

ECHR. (2016). *Case of Wenner v Germany*. https://hudoc.echr.coe.int/eng#{%22fulltext%22:[%2262303/13%22],%22documentcollectionid2%22:[%22GRANDCHAMBER%22,%22CHAMBER%22],%22itemid%22:[%22001–165758%22]}

Flanagan, J. (2022). *Embedding a new model of care in addiction nursing: How one team's journey influenced behaviours & practices across wider frontiers*. Retrieved February 26, 2024 from https://healthservice.hse.ie/filelibrary/onmsd/embedding-a-new-model-of-care-in-addiction-nursing-jean-flanagan.pdf

Goldberg, D. (1978). *Manual of the general health questionnaire*. NFER-Nelson.

Health Service Executive. (2023). *Partnership principles. Building a new relationship between voluntary organisations and the State in the health and social care sectors*. rep. Available at: https://www.lenus.ie/handle/10147/641371?show=full. Accessed 03 June 2024.

Holland, A., Harris, M., Hickman, M., Lewer, D., Shorter, G.W., Horsley, J., Powell, M., Rae, M. (2022). Overdose prevention centres in the UK. *The Lancet Public Health, 7*(3), e196–e197, https://doi.org/10.1016/S2468-2667(22)00038-X. (https://www.sciencedirect.com/science/article/pii/S246826672200038X)

INCB. (2019). *International Narcotics Control Board, Annual Reports, Thematic Chapters 1*. Retrieved February 22, 2024 from https://www.incb.org/incb/en/publications/annual-reports/annual-report.html

INCB. (2020). *International Narcotics Control Board, Annual Reports, Thematic Chapters 1*. Retrieved February 22, 2024 from https://www.incb.org/incb/en/publications/annual-reports/annual-report.html

INCB. (2021). *International Narcotics Control Board, Annual Reports, Thematic Chapters 1*. Retrieved February 22, 2024 from https://www.incb.org/incb/en/publications/annual-reports/annual-report.html

INCB. (2022). *International Narcotics Control Board, Annual Reports, Thematic Chapters 1*. Retrieved February 22, 2024 from https://www.incb.org/incb/en/publications/annual-reports/annual-report.html

INCB. (2023). *International Narcotics Control Board, Annual Reports, Thematic Chapters 1*. Retrieved February 22, 2024 from https://www.incb.org/incb/en/publications/annual-reports/annual-report.html

Institute for Capacity Strengthening. (2015). *Partnership approaches, Catholic relief services*. Available at: https://ics.crs.org/partnership-approaches. Accessed: 03 June 2024.

Jaffe, J. (2000). *Frontline: Interview with Jerome Jaffe Response to question: How did the moralizing of the drug issue affect treatment?* Retrieved March 22, 2024 from https://www.pbs.org/wgbh/pages/frontline/shows/drugs/interviews/jaffe.html

Leahy-Warren, P., Mulcahy, H., Benefield, L., Bradley, C., Coffey, A., Donohoe, A., Fitzgerald, S., Frawley, T., Healy, E., & Healy, M. (2017). Conceptualising a model to guide nursing and midwifery in the community guided by an evidence review. *BMC Nursing, 16*, 1–13.

Marder, I. (2024). Embedding a culture of interdisciplinary open research in criminal justice in Ireland: Agreeing purposes and principles for the criminal justice open research dialogue (CORD) partnership. *Irish Probation Journal*.

McCorry, F., Garnick, D. W., Bartlett, J., Cotter, F., Chalk, M., Babor, T., Falcon, S., Gastfriend, D. R., Gelber, S., & Harrison, P. A. (2000). Developing performance measures for alcohol and other drug services in managed care plans. *The Joint Commission Journal on Quality Improvement, 26*(11), 633–643.

O'Neill, D., De Vries, J., & Comiskey, C. M. (2021). Leadership and community healthcare reform: A study using the competing values framework (CVF). *Leadership in Health Services, 34*(4), 485–498.

Pompidou Group. (2024). *Children whose parents use drugs*. Council of Europe Portal. Retrieved February 28, 2024 from https://www.coe.int/en/web/pompidou/children

Razaghi, E., Binazadeh, M., Negarandeh, R., & Bradford, J. (2023). The hidden aspects of a century of substance use policymaking in Iran. *Qeios*. https://doi.org/10.32388/Q0PMCL

Robin, M. (1969). *The French Connection*. Little, Brown, and Company (Boston, United States ISBN 1-59228- 044-7

Sterling, M. (2011). General health questionnaire–28 (GHQ-28). *Journal of Physiotherapy, 57*(4), 259.

Strang, J. (2011). *Recovery-orientated drug treatment: An interim report*. National Treatment Agency. Retrieved February 26, 2024 from https://www.drugsandalcohol.ie/15524/1/NTA_Strand_recovery_oriented.pdf

Tang, H., Li, M., Yan, X., Lu, Z., & Jia, Z. (2021). Modeling the dynamics of drug spreading in China. *International Journal of Environmental Research and Public Health, 18*(1), 288. https://doi.org/10.3390/ijerph18010288

UN. (1966). *International Covenant on Economic, Social and Cultural Rights*, United Nations, New York, USA. Retrieved April 24, 2020 from https://www.ohchr.org/EN/ProfessionalInterest/Pages/CESCR.aspx

UN. (1979, December 18). *Convention on the elimination of all forms of discrimination against women New York*. United Nations. Retrieved April 27, 2020 from https://www.ohchr.org/en/professionalinterest/pages/cedaw.aspx

UN. (1989, November 20). *Convention on the rights of the child*. Retrieved March 11, 2019 from https://www.refworld.org/docid/3ae6b38f0.html

UN. (2016, December 12). *Secretary-General-designate António Guterres' remarks to the General Assembly on taking the oath of office*. Retrieved April 4, 2024 from https://www.un.org/sg/en/content/sg/speeches/2016-12-12/secretary-general-designate-ant%C3%B3nio-guterres-oath-office-speech

United Nations (UNGASS). (2016). *Outcome document of the 2016 united nations general Assembly special session on the world drug problem*. available at Outcome document of the thirtieth special session 19-21 April 2016 (citywide.ie) Accessed February 20th 2024.

UN Sustainable Development Group. (2016). *Applying foresight and alternative futures to the United Nations development assistance framework*. Retrieved November 29, 2023, from https://unsdg.un.org/resources/applying-foresight-and-alternative-futures-united-nations-development-assistance

Yang, J., & Giummarra, M. J. (2021). Compulsory and voluntary drug treatment models in China: A need for improved evidence-based policy and practice to reduce the loaded burden of substance use disorders. *International Journal of Drug Policy, 92*, 103063.

Chapter 10
Implementation, Monitoring, and Evaluation: What Enablers Do We Need and When Do We Need Them to Ensure Success?

Setting the Scene

Steve Jobs on failure, measurement, and implementation:

> *In order to learn how to do something well, you have to fail sometimes. In order to fail, there has to be a measurement system. And that's the problem with most philanthropy – there's no measurement system. You give somebody some money to do something and most of the time you can really never measure whether you failed or succeeded in your judgment of that person or his ideas or their implementation. (Jobs,* 1985*)*

Introduction

Despite its reputation for notoriety, *Playboy* magazine included a range of memorable interviews with leaders such as Martin Luther King Jr., Stanley Kubrick, Bette Davis, Miles Davis, and Steve Jobs among others. The quote above is from Jobs' lengthy interview with journalist David Sheff. The interview was conducted approximately 40 years ago in 1985. This was in the early days of the Internet, and it was the year that Jobs was forced out of Apple. In the interview Jobs speaks of his initial steps into philanthropy. As can be seen from his words, in terms of his charity he clearly notes his misgivings about a lack of measurement and a lack of implementation. To enable resources to be appropriately expended, there is a need to ensure that monitoring, evaluation, and implementation are adequately addressed within an intervention's rollout be that a policy, a service, or a new practice.

The gap between what is known from research, to applying that research in real-life situations is referred to as the "implementation gap." This gap is often humorously referred to in "mind the gap" illustrations or in mathematically complex illustrations with gaps stating a miracle occurs to achieve the final result (see Wade (2016) for an illustration). We often unwittingly expect this miracle to occur and our

C. Comiskey, *Addiction Research and Evaluation*, Advances in Mental Health and Addiction, https://doi.org/10.1007/978-3-031-65917-1_10

new policy, new service improvement plan or new intervention will be successfully rolled out and operationalized. Unfortunately, experience has told us that this is seldom the case.

Implementation science has developed as a discipline to address this gap between science and practice. It seeks to understand and map the processes to take what is known from scientific evidence and to bring this evidence to inform and improve policy and practice. Implementation science can be defined as:

> *the study of the process of implementing programs and practices that have some evidence from the research field to suggest they are worth replicating. It is the study of how a practice that is evidence-based or evidence-informed gets translated to different, more diverse contexts in the real world. (Metz* et al., 2015, *p. 1).*

Burke et al. (2012) state that at its simplest implementation can be described as the carrying out of a plan for doing something. That something could be the introduction of a new evidence-based program or intervention or way of working into a new context, such as a different practice or service. Implementation can be the carrying out of the actions of a new policy's objectives and goals or it can be the introduction of a process of quality improvement steps. Implementation can refer to any innovation.

Implementation science focuses on the strategies that can promote implementation success and the theoretical underpinnings of these strategies. Eccles and Mittman (2006) in their opening editorial of a new implementation science journal for the emerging discipline recognized the gap and noted that research findings were not leading to changes in outcomes and that this would not change unless health services and professionals adopted the findings into practice. The journal pioneered implementation research and they stated that:

> *Implementation research is the scientific study of methods to promote the systematic uptake of research findings and other evidence-based practices into routine practice, and, hence, to improve the quality and effectiveness of health services. It includes the study of influences on healthcare professional and organisational behaviour. Eccles and Mittman* (2006, *p. 1).*

The literature in the discipline of implementation science has developed and expanded. It has built on the significant body of knowledge and research from a range of related disciplines including management, change management, and organizational development.

Implementation Science Frameworks

Wang et al. (2023) provide a scoping review of implementation science theories, models, and frameworks (TMFs). They examined 143 theories, models and frameworks and concluded that the usability of these needs to be improved. They noted that little attention was paid to the wider contexts, stages of scale-up and sustainability and implementation outcomes such as feasibility, cost, and penetration. There was also a lack of recommended measurement methods to all to the TMFs.

The United States, National Institute of Health (NIH, 2023) drawing on an earlier review of Moullin et al. (2015) and Nilsen (2020) presents a summary of five frameworks, two of which are presented here due to their frequent use. A third developed by Burke et al. (2012) is also presented given its ease of use in a broad range of settings.

The RE-AIM Framework and PRISM

The RE-AIM framework of Glasgow et al. (1999) is considered more operational than others and involves both dissemination and implementation issues. It considers the interaction between five factors; these are summarized in Table 10.1.

Further information is available at (RE-AIM, 2024) where details of the framework are provided. In addition, information on the related PRISM tool is provided. PRISM is the **P**ractical **R**obust **I**mplementation **S**ustainability **M**odel. PRISM includes RE-AIM but it is wider as it includes contextual factors that are important as a program, policy or practice is implemented within varying settings. PRISM explores perspectives from multiple sectors or stakeholders. It looks at the external environment, including recognizing inequities. It explores partner characteristics and finally it explores the infrastructure available for implementation and ongoing sustainability.

The Consolidated Framework for Implementation Research (CFIR)

Damschroder et al. (2009) noted that many theories had been published to help promote effective implementation. While the theories can overlap, when the theories were compared each was found to be missing a key construct. The Consolidated

Table 10.1 A summary of the five factors of the RE-AIM framework

Reach	This is an individual level measure of participation and refers to the percentage and risk characteristics of persons who receive or are affected by a policy or program
Effectiveness	Effectiveness refers to the individual-level change in the primary outcome, impact on quality of life, and assessment of potential negative outcomes resulting from the intervention
Adoption	Adoption refers the proportion and representativeness of settings that adopt a given policy or program
Implementation	Implementation means the extent to which a program is delivered as intended
Maintenance	Maintenance measures the extent to which innovations become a relatively stable, enduring part of the behavioral repertoire of an individual, organization, or community

Framework for Implementation Research (CFIR) was developed and presents an overarching typology to promote implementation theory development and verification about what works where and why across multiple contexts. Damschroder et al. (2009) found that while many interventions were effective, in health services research studies they failed to translate into improved outcomes when applied across multiple and varying contexts. There was a need not just for summative evaluations but also formative ones to inform efficacy in specific settings and prolong sustainability. The CFIR was developed and is composed of five major domains each supported by varying constructs as summarized in Table 10.2.

According to the CFIR developers, researchers should assess each construct for importance and relevance to their work. Operational definitions of the constructs should be formed in accordance with the study application and some constructs may overlap. The level of measurement at which the constructs should be evaluated also needs to be considered. Some may be at an individual level and others at a team or service level. It is also important to note that the long list of constructs may not be needed for each implementation study.

The Centre for Effective Services (CES) Framework

Burke et al. (2012) address the practical challenges for services trying to navigate the literature on varying frameworks and provide an excellent introductory guide to implementation science. They summarize the stages of implementation identified by Fixsen (2005). These are illustrated in Fig. 10.1.

During the exploring and preparing stage there are some excellent tools that can be used to explore the factors that need to be assessed before adopting and implementing an innovation. The Hexagon Tool developed by the National Implementation Research Network (Metz & Louison, 2019) can be used to assess the suitability of an innovation for the organization, the setting and the context. If an innovation is deemed suitable then organizational readiness for change (ORC) can be assessed. Simpson (2009) have developed a comprehensive ORC survey that can be used by addiction services to help them in this process. Finally, Burke et al. (2012) provide a simple listing of enablers across the stage of implementation. This list can be used by services as a checklist to identify resources and actions that they may need to address to aid their implementation. Table 10.3 summarizes these enablers. The Department of Health (2018) provides further details for clinical guidelines implementation.

In terms of building upon monitoring and evaluation and learning from experience the use of Plan Do Study Act Cycles (PDSA) to aid continuous improvement can be very useful. Reflecting on the outcomes of the implementation process can lead to improved insights on where further changes or supports are needed (Department of Health, 2018). Figure 10.2 illustrates this process.

Table 10.2 A summary of the five domains and underlying construct in the Consolidated Framework for Implementation Research (CFIR) based on Damschroder et al. (2009)

Intervention characteristics	Intervention source. Evidence strength and quality. Relative advantage. Adaptability. Trialability. Complexity. Design quality and packaging. Cost.
Outer setting	Patient needs and resources. Cosmopolitanism. Peer pressure. External policies and incentives.
Inner setting	Structural characteristics. Networks and communications. Culture. Implementation climate: Six sub-constructs contribute to a positive implementation climate for an intervention: Tension for change, compatibility, relative priority, organizational incentives and rewards, goals and feedback, and learning climate. Readiness for implementation with three sub-constructs (leadership engagement, available resources, and access to information and knowledge).
Characteristics of the individuals involved	Knowledge and beliefs about the intervention. Self-efficacy. Individual stage of change. Individual identification with organization. Other personal attributes.
The process of implementation	Planning. Engaging. Executing and reflecting. Evaluating.

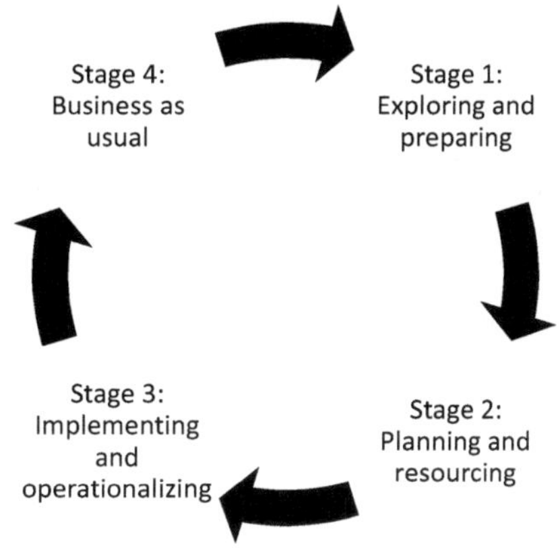

Fig. 10.1 The four stages of implementation

Table 10.3 Identifying barriers and a checklist of enablers and when they are needed across the stages of implementation. (Adapted from Burke et al., 2012)

Enablers	Stage of implementation			
	1. Exploring and preparing	**2. Planning and resourcing**	**3. Implementing and operationalizing**	**4. Business as usual**
Leadership	✓	✓	✓	✓
Resources	✓	✓	✓	✓
Stakeholder consultation and buy-in	✓	✓	✓	✓
Supportive organizational culture		✓	✓	✓
Organizational support		✓	✓	✓
Implementation plan		✓	✓	✓
Implementation teams		✓	✓	✓
Staff capacity		✓	✓	✓
Communication		✓	✓	✓
Monitoring and evaluation			✓	✓
Learning from experience			✓	✓
Barriers across the implementation stages	External environment; resistance to change; vested interests			

The Generic Implementation Framework (GIF)

Moullin et al. (2015) present what they term the Generic Implementation Framework (GIF). The GIF depicts the core concepts of implementation. It highlights the non-linear and recursive nature of the implementation process. The process is also divided into a series of stages and/or steps. At the center of the framework is the innovation/policy/practice to be implemented and surrounding the innovation are the contextual domains or levels of influence. Throughout the process, at each stage and for each domain, there are factors, strategies, and evaluations that will influence the outcome of the implementation. The GIF is not a new framework but rather a compilation of what is represented in most, other frameworks. Using the GIF as a checklist can help ensure that the detailed framework(s) chosen for the implementation cover the core implementation concepts. Table 10.4 provides an adapted visual of the GIF.

Fig. 10.2 The Plan Do Study Act (PDSA) continuous improvement cycle for use in implementation

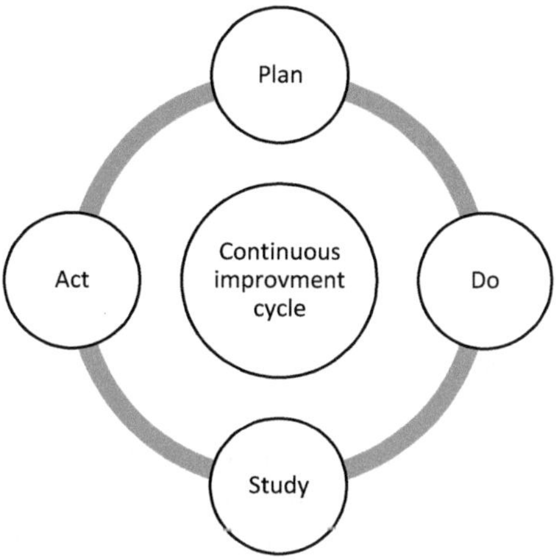

Selecting a Framework

When selecting a framework to implement an innovation Moullin et al. (2015) following their systematic review suggest that the study group should ensure all concepts are covered. To do this they may have to select a range of frameworks. They highlight that the concepts that should be considered include those relating to the process of implementation (the stages and steps), the innovation to be implemented, the context in which the implementation is to occur (divided into various numbers of domains), influencing factors, strategies, and evaluations.

For example, they state that an organization wanting to implement a program may need to use a more prescriptive framework that spans all the implementation stages as well as being particularly detailed on strategies and evaluations. Alternatively, a researcher conducting an implementation study may wish to focus primarily on the overarching concept of implementation, e.g., on the factors affecting implementation, and therefore the Consolidated Framework for Implementation Research could be suitable.

Moullin et al. (2015) notes that following their review they found that it is often the case that implementation frameworks, models, and theories are not created to be holistic, but rather target a specific implementation concept, such as a stage, or either the factors, strategies, or evaluations. Consequently, if an inclusive implementation framework is required, an alternative to selecting a comprehensive, holistic innovation-specific framework might be to choose a combination of frameworks to cover the depth of each element.

Table 10.4 An adapted presentation of the generic implementation framework (GIF)

Pre-implementation	Process of implementation	Post-implementation
Strategies, factors and evaluations		
The innovation/policy/practice/service		
The context domains		

Fidelity

Fidelity is the degree to which the activities undertaken in a program (or intervention, policy, or practice) are true to the design of the original program on which it is based (Burke et al., 2012). It is the degree to which an intervention was delivered as it was intended to be. Other terms used include, delivered as intended; adherence; integrity; and finally, quality of delivery. There can however be a tension between the need to ensure fidelity and the need to adapt to a changing setting or environment. In real-life settings and applications, it is unlikely that an implementation plan, for example, will be implemented with 100% fidelity. Challenges and alteration in timing and roll out can and will be experienced.

Where caution must be exercised is in the core components of an intervention. For example, if sufficient timing isn't allocated to identifying the local needs and establishing buy-in then a previously successful program can underperform. This challenge was found when implementing a healthy school's program among urban disadvantaged schools. Comiskey et al. (2015) in their evaluation found that the program manual wasn't available for schools that had enrolled in the program. The checklist for identifying local needs wasn't completed. As a result, the outcomes for children and the school were slow to change.

McGilloway (2009) in a pragmatic randomized control trial in a community setting of the Incredible Years Parenting Program ensured that parents received all the training involved in the program manual. Consequently, they ensured that fidelity to the program was followed by supporting parents to attend the program with child minding provided and funding for travel supplied. Parenting skills were found to improve as expected and child behavioral challenges were lessened.

When implementing a program, the measure of fidelity is essential to understand why or why not a program may or may not have performed as expected.

Monitoring and Evaluation

The Organization for Economic Co-operation and Development known as the OECD was established over 60 years ago and aims to create better polices for better lives. With the involvement of governments, policy makers and citizens they focus on establishing and sharing evidence-based international standards and developing solutions to a range of social, economic, and environmental challenges. To date they have 38 member countries and many partners. Members span North and South America to Europe and the Asia-Pacific region. Key partners include Brazil, China, India, Indonesia, and South Africa. Regional initiatives span Africa, Eurasia, the Middle East and North Africa, Latin America and the Caribbean, Southeast Asia, and Southeast Europe (OECD, 2023). Given the overarching OECD aim, monitoring and evaluation is a central part of their work to support policy with scientific evidence.

The Independent Evaluation Group of the World Bank cites the OECD definitions of monitoring and evaluation. Monitoring the state can be defined as:

> *A continuing function that uses systematic collection of data on specified indicators to provide management and the main stakeholders of an ongoing development intervention with indications of the extent of progress and achievement of objectives and progress in the use of allocated funds. (IEG,* 2024*).*

We can see from this definition that monitoring is continuous and that systematic data collection is used to assist stakeholders in the measurement of the progress of objectives within an intervention, policy, practice, or service. Monitoring on its own is, however, not sufficient, as the data generated is limited to a set of indicators. One of the key roles of monitoring is to contribute to evaluations.

Evaluation the IEG (2024) define as, "*the process of determining the worth or significance of a development activity, policy or program .. to determine the relevance of objectives, the efficacy of design and implementation, the efficiency or resource use, and the sustainability of results. An evaluation should (enable) the incorporation of lessons learned into the decision-making process of both partner and donor*." They state that monitoring and evaluation are synergistic, they work together to provide better information. Evaluation can provide a more balanced interpretation of performance indicators collected during the monitoring process. Evaluation is more time-consuming and while monitoring is continuous, evaluation is conducted not continuously but regularly at appropriate intervals.

The EMCDDA (2021) in their action framework for health and social responses highlight that monitoring, evaluation, and feedback are essential for good service delivery. This depends upon the establishment of sustainable data collection systems. If the data is to be useful then it needs to be routinely collected and be complete. The feedback loop enables staff to assess their progress on what is working for whom and where. Perhaps even more importantly the monitoring, evaluation, and feedback can highlight any unforeseen negative consequences, and this is essential to ensure a new intervention, policy or practice is meeting its aims and objectives while doing no harm. A failure to monitor and evaluate is a failure to provide good governance.

Developing a Monitoring and Evaluation System

Kusek and Rist (2004) in their handbook for development practitioners of the World Bank, provide a succinct booklet outlining ten steps for the development of a results-based monitoring and evaluation system. While their applications relate to country level implementations the steps remain relevant within different contexts and settings. Kusek and Rist (2004) provide additional details within the steps that can be used to guide their completion. These ten steps are outlined in Fig. 10.3.

Step 1, readiness for change has been discussed previously. The importance of agreeing outcomes across stakeholders is essential in step 2. Varying stakeholders can advise on what is both feasible and useful within their context and ensuring their buy-in and contribution to the decision-making process is necessary for both success and sustainability. The selecting of key performance indicators from the monitoring data should aim to encompass measures to assess progress spanning the setting. For example, within the European Monitoring Centre for Drugs and Drug Addiction (EMCDDA) five key epidemiological indicators were established. These were, the prevalence of drug use within the general population, the prevalence of problem drug use, the number of deaths, the numbers of Hepatitis C and HIV cases and finally the treatment demand indicator. We can see from these five that they reflect a broad span of needs at varying population levels and key treatment levels.

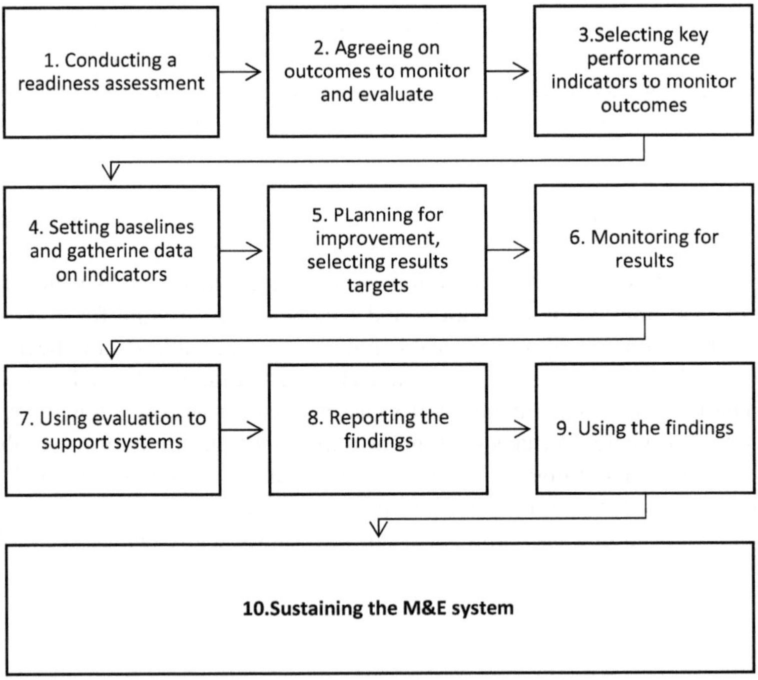

Fig. 10.3 The ten steps for developing a monitoring and evaluation system. (Adapted from Kusek and Rist, 2004)

To assess progress, within step 4 it is essential that baseline data is gathered from which changes can be measured. This includes both improvements and any unintended consequences. For example, implementing tighter controls on opioid pain medications availability to reduce diversions may increase accessibility to that medication for those suffering or people at end-of-life care. Step 5 requires organizations to set realistic targets and again this should be done in consultation with stakeholders. A realistic target for the treatment demand indicator of the EMCDDA could be that anyone who requires treatment is provided with that treatment within a defined time. Given local treatment systems this duration could be 1 month in some locations or 1 week or 1 day in others. This example illustrates the need for consultation on feasibility with local stakeholders. Step 6 is the establishment of the monitoring system to enable the work. There are two aspects to this, the monitoring of the implementation and the monitoring of the results. Monitoring of results will not be achieved if the system is not implemented as planned.

Step 7 addresses evaluation and their use to support decision-making and evaluating progress. There are different types of approaches and methods to evaluation and these details are discussed in a separate section. One key aspect of evaluation is the timing and the choice of when to evaluate. While this is a simple question to answer it requires an in-depth knowledge of the application and the setting. For example, within opiate agonist treatment it is known that reductions in illicit opioid use occur very quickly and often within the first month of treatment. However, improvements in mental well-being may take far longer for some people (Gossop et al., 2000). Reporting the findings and feeding back in an accessible and useful way to the target audience is a key step in the plan do study act cycles. This feedback will enable the findings to be used to improve the overall monitoring and evaluation system and will identify where modifications or potentially resources are most needed.

Sustaining a Monitoring and Evaluation System

To sustain a monitoring and evaluation (M&E) system, there must be demand and use for the data generated. One key additional added value of the data generated, apart from the use of the data by stakeholders to improve the policy/practice/service for staff and clients, is the evidence the monitoring and evaluation generates. This independent objective evidence can be used to identify key needs and negotiate for resources for those needs.

An M&E system will not be sustained if clear roles and responsibilities for it are not allocated and given dedicated time and resources. The data arising from the system will not be trusted or may be seen to only be partially representative if the system is not audited for completeness and accuracy. Accountability for the system is distributed across all those involved in the system and leadership and good governances of the system are essential. To enable staff to assume and take this accountability there must be capacity within the staff and the resources and adequate training must be provided for both the technical, operational, and administrative aspects of the system. One incentive to ensure staff buy-in is the visibility of how the M&E system assists with providing the evidence for both staff and client needs and how this can be translated into extra resources being allocated on a fair and equitable basis.

Conducting an Evaluation

Conducting an evaluation is a team effort that may involve additional expertise in evaluation design and execution. A listing of key steps in conducting an evaluation were first detailed by the Centre for Disease Control and Prevention in 1999 (CDC, 1999). An online summary of the steps including a supporting checklist is now available (CDC, 2021). These steps are provided in Fig. 10.4.

Quite often resources will not allow for a full program evaluation and while in step 2 the full program may be described it is within step 3 that the focus of the evaluation and its resulting design will be decided. This decision should include the four key standards of evaluation, these being:

1. Utility: Who has the greatest need for this evaluation and how will they use it?
2. Feasibility: If those areas with greatest need have been identified is there the feasibility to conduct an evaluation in this area. Is the money, time, skill, and resources available?
3. Propriety: For inclusivity, diversity, and ethics, who needs to be involved in the evaluation? For example, are clients involved and if so, is their involvement ethical and supported?
4. Accuracy: Is the chosen design appropriate, will it provide the right information?

The choice of evaluation design should reflect the focus of the evaluation and the four key standards. A summary of designs is provided in Table 10.5.

The design of outcome evaluations can be experimental (a randomized control trial, for example, with an intervention and a control group randomly assigned).

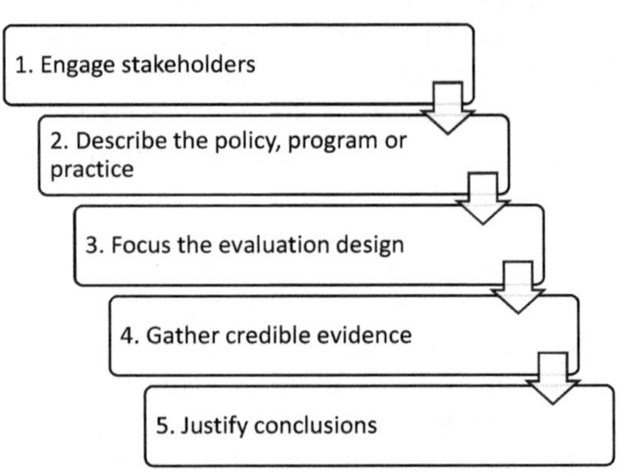

Fig. 10.4 Outline of the five key steps in evaluation. (Adapted from CDC, 2021)

Table 10.5 A summary of evaluation designs and their roles

Types of evaluations				
Formative	Summative	Process	Outcomes	Impact
These evaluate an intervention (policy, program or service) during its development with the aim of making improvements relevant to the context.	These are conducted after an intervention has been designed. They aim to provide information on its effectiveness.	Process evaluations focus on the implementation to assess if the intervention was rolled out as intended and with fidelity.	Outcome evaluations measure changes in directly relevant measures before and after the roll out of the intervention.	Impact evaluations focus on measuring longer-term sustainability of changes because of the intervention.

Adapted from the Peak Performance Centre (2024)

They can be quasi-experimental with both an intervention and a comparison group without randomization. Or the outcome evaluation can be nonexperimental with pre- and post-measurements. Nonexperimental designs are used when it unethical to use a nonintervention group, for example when one cannot deny a treatment for substance use. In these situations, pre- and post-measures are usually taken within the intervention group. Several other evaluation types exist for different situations. For example, there are several types of economic evaluations but these are beyond the scope of this chapter.

Potential Methods for Evaluation Data Collection

Data collection approaches fall primarily into two types: qualitative methods and quantitative ones. Qualitative methods can include observation, which can be structured, semi-structured or unstructured. Structured observation usually requires a checklist and specific items are noted in the observation. To ensure all evaluators involved in the observational data collection are observing correctly either in the structured or nonstructured approach, all should be trained and then a pilot test should be completed to assess findings and inter-observer reliability. A good example of this was conducted in the Incredible Years Parenting Program (McGilloway et al., 2009). All observers of parental behaviors were trained to observe both positive and negative parental reactions used with a young child with conduct disorder challenges.

Observing meetings and how they are conducted can also be a useful data source, as can be meeting minutes. Banka Cullen et al. (2022) in the DAVINA project observed facilitators working with women who use drugs and who were co-creating an anti-stigma training program for statutory service providers. Observers took a semi-structured approach observing set indicators of power imbalance but also noting other aspects such as the room layout, placement of materials and levels of participation of group members.

Meeting minutes and other written communications such as emails, printed materials, notice boards, can all be used to observe the adherence to the stated value systems of an organization. This approach was used by Comiskey et al. (2018) when evaluating a gay men's health outreach program. Similarly online screen grabs of text messages can be used to observe service values and delivery of eHealth and mHealth initiatives. Other novel qualitative methods include visual and construction methods, such as drawings, photovoice, video, Lego serious play and performance.

Standard qualitative approaches include focus groups which allow interaction among participants and can stimulate broader responses and more in-depth responses to some topics. With focus groups it is important to have both a facilitator and a supportive observer who can intervene to support the facilitator if they observe that some focus group members are reluctant to engage.

One-on-one interviews when conducted correctly with a trained interviewer can provide in-depth personal responses to sensitive topics that can only be addressed by an individual. The disadvantage is that only one viewpoint is obtained. Several one-on-one interviews with varying individuals are often required. If the interviewer is not prepared or trained, then the depth of the interview responses can be compromised, and perfunctory responses can be obtained. The interview schedule can also be structured, semi-structured or unstructured. However even with a structured interview it can be worthwhile to allow the interviewee the scope to expand on a topic and new insights can be gained.

Quantitative methods are also very varied and include existing record systems. These have the advantage in that they are already in place, but they may be limited by a lack of consistency in record keeping or they may have a lack of relevant data. Records can be at the individual level or at a service level. The quantitative indicators developed for the monitoring system can be used for the evaluation. These will provide retrospective data. These retrospective records may be paper based on computer data-based.

Similarly innovative data capture methods can be employed and downloaded from online systems for eHealth and mHealth. These can provide ongoing current data: this can be system usage data including potentially video and audio data. Data scrapping techniques of online systems and platforms can also be used.

Traditional quantitative data methods such as surveys can also be harnessed, and these can be face-to-face paper-based survey interviews or supported live online surveys or anonymous online surveys. With these surveys it is important to ensure participants contribute only once, unless the evaluation design allows for repeated survey measurements over a period of time.

To conclude, the monitoring and indicator data, alongside the myriad of other potential data collection methods, provides a wealth of information that can be used for evaluation. Furthermore, evaluators should seek to use a mix of both traditional and novel approaches to ensure all appropriate voices and opinions are included.

Case Study 10.1: Using the Centre for Effective Services (CES) Framework to Evaluate the Implementation of an Education Program in South Africa

Introduction

Globally there is a recognized shortage of nursing and other healthcare professionals educated at baccalaureate level and beyond. Nickitas and Feeg (2011) found that less than 1% of nurses have a doctoral degree and predicted that there will be significant shortfalls in future nurse academics, and nurse practitioners. This shortage is most acute in low- to middle-income countries. Many countries are addressing these shortages in healthcare provision by ensuring that the basic nursing education qualification is at degree level. They are also developing advanced nursing roles which have a wider remit and which require research degrees. Within South Africa there have been policies to address education capacity development and inequity in healthcare while simultaneously, the healthcare system has been dealing with substantial numbers of people with HIV/AIDS, unprecedented violence and crime-related injuries and substance use (Sheehan et al., 2015). Within the South African educational system, the PhD Proposal Development Program for Nursing Sciences, was developed from a collaborative international knowledge network that included Doctoral Candidates of Nursing Sciences, Supervisors/Promoters, Universities, Development Partners and an implementing organization called SANTRUST. This was an educational trust that contributed to doctoral education and capacity development since 1997 (Smit et al., 2013).

The PhD development program involved 23 universities from across South Africa, their nursing PhD candidates and their supervisors. The program consisted of six modules, each delivered face to face over a single week. The six modules were held consecutively and completed over the course of an academic year. All six modules were compulsory and were attended by the nurses undertaking the proposal development stage of their PhD. While much was expected of the program, the primary impact expected was an increased PhD capacity within the universities. The primary outcome measure was the successful completion of the PhD at an individual level. To learn from the SANTRUST experience and to assess the program's implementation and outcomes, an evaluation of the program was conducted.

Methods

To evaluate the implementation of the SANTRUST program, the implementation framework of Burke et al. (2012) was applied. Participants in the evaluation included 55 students who participated in the program over two cohorts from admission to completion of the program, program facilitators (lecturers and tutors), and program staff (program managers and administrators). A range of data sources were accessed including the funding proposal, the curriculum for the program, regular evaluation reports from the nursing PhD program participants and program facilitators, meeting notes, and finally, measurable outcome indicators on PhD candidate retention and successful completion rates. Ethical approval was not required as all data was openly available within evaluation reports from candidates and annual reports. In addition, the evaluation statistics were regularly fed back to the candidates who had participated in them.

As the CES framework was used to guide the evaluation, a deductive, top-down approach was used to analyze the data. Evidence within the data sources for each of the implementation enablers and barriers was sought and then mapped onto the framework.

Results

Table 10.6 provides an excerpt of the findings mapped onto the framework. From this we can clearly see where across the stages of implementation there was either evidence or lack thereof of a known enabler. For example, within staff capacity at stage 2, program staff were recruited but at stage 3 during implementing and operationalizing, supervisors were failing to attend their module in the program. Monitoring and evaluation was found to be well implemented but resources while sufficient for the program were not sustainable, as can be seen in stage 4. In terms of barriers evidence was found to support the key barriers of resistance to change, vested interests and external environmental factors.

Discussion

The CES framework provided an excellent tool to map and visualize, in a meaningful way for stakeholders, the presence and staging challenges to the enablers of successful implementation. The monitoring of key indicators on retention and completion rates provided direct measurable evidence of expected outcomes from the program. This evidence could then be enhanced by the findings from the framework, which clearly demonstrated that the program worked. It was however not sustainable in its current format and funding model. Without additional buy-in from those universities resistant to change, perhaps due to vested interests or the funding environment available to them, the program while fit for purpose needed to be adapted to the environment to remain viable.

To conclude the implementation science approach, the framework and the quantitative and qualitative data collection methods were extremely useful in providing evidence that can be easily shared and interpreted by those with the power to effect change within the internal barriers and the broader systemic issues.

Table 10.6 An excerpt of findings on implementation enablers across the stages of a nursing PhD capacity development program. (Adapted from Sheehan et al., 2015)

Enablers	Stage of implementation			
	Stage 1 Exploring and preparing	Stage 2 Planning and resourcing	Stage 3 Implementation and operation	Stage 4 Business as usual
Resources	Support by SANPAD and existing SANTRUST program; funding proposal developed for Irish aid. Support from Irish aid and NRF given in principle.	Funding secured for pilot stage from Irish AID for 2012–2013; CFO hired and financial and logistical support outsourced; national and international academics recruited to deliver program.	Additional funding secured for 2013–2014. Evaluation committee set up to select doctoral candidates against call criteria; A second program manager was appointed. Constraints in obtaining co-financing from universities.	The final cohort became fully funded without co-financing from universities, due to savings on previous programs, but this is unlikely to be repeated.
Staff capacity		Program staff recruited according to the skills and needs for the operation of the program; all facilitators selected were vetted for appropriate skill and experience mix.	A PhD supervisors module was embedded to build supervisory capacity but has not been well attended. Candidates take learning back to their organizations and faculties and apply double-loop learning.	Candidates continue to take their learning back to their organizations and faculties.
Monitoring and evaluation			Written feedback obtained from candidates, facilitators, supervisors, and reviewers after Every module (reviewed by evaluation Committee); internal monitoring against Strategy during staff meetings.	Standard practice of modular reporting continues.

Case Study 10.2: Using the Consolidated Framework for Implementation Research to Evaluate a Research Program in a Hospital and Its HIV/AIDS Clinic

Introduction

Nursing participation in research is low and in addiction research it is lower. This is despite nursing professionals working daily with relevant clients and data, which could be used to generate evidence for their practice and their patients. Within the more advanced nursing roles, one of the competencies includes research. There is now an expectancy that advanced nursing staff will be research active and undertake research.

Given this expectation there is clearly a need, not only to provide research capacity development and ongoing support, but also to evaluate its effectiveness (McKee et al., 2017). The aim of this project was to describe the implementation of an intervention and evaluate its effectiveness in increasing research capacity in advanced clinical nursing roles and to illustrate this with an example from the hospitals HIV clinic (Farrell & Comiskey, 2014).

According to McKee et al. (2017), the intervention included a series of tripartite groupings of a the clinical nurse, an academic nurse with related research interests to the clinical setting and a facilitator in the form of a postdoctoral researcher. The intervention developed included, skill development, support with quantitative methodology and support from the additional researchers experienced in both carrying out research and research dissemination.

The key characteristics of the intervention were leadership, a steering group, funding, the small research groups with the postdoctoral support and focused clinical nurse-led research questions. Funding was sourced to employ a part-time postdoctoral researcher who had both quantitative and health research experience. This postdoctoral researcher acted as a research facilitator and provided both expertise and sharing of research workload with the clinical and academic nurse researchers. Through the utilization of the skills of both clinical and academic partners the intervention aimed to facilitate the understanding, development, and application of research skills, to produce demonstrable outputs for patient care and research.

Methods

The Consolidated Framework for Implementation Research (CFIR) was used to underpin the evaluation. A mixed methods design with quantitative and qualitative data sources were analyzed. All staff in advanced nursing roles were invited to take part in the intervention and those who were interested and who had a potential project participated. Data for the evaluation was generated from focus groups and a survey of skills. Indicators measuring the number of successful research outputs generated were measured. The CFIR was used to aid the reporting of the findings in terms of the characteristics of the intervention, the outer or environmental/social context of the intervention, the inner setting or local context, the characteristics of the participants and the process.

Results

Details of the findings in relation to the framework are provided in McKee et al. (2017). In summary in terms of outcomes and indicators, in the first year, 12 new clinical nurse-led research projects were conducted and reported in eight peer-reviewed papers, two non-peer-reviewed papers and 15 conference presentations.

One of these papers was the findings, hitherto unreported, on patients attending the HIV/AIDS clinic who also had a dual diagnosis of Hepatitis C and were ineligible or nonresponsive to treatment. The research undertaken by the nurse running the clinic uncovered that her patients experienced not only the duality of infection but the duality of fear and hope, rejection and acceptance and moving from feelings of death to looking forward to unexpected futures. This project's output from the larger intervention went on to be internationally published and also presented within a global podcast for nurses working with HIV/AIDS patients (Farrell & Comiskey, 2014).

Discussion

The main strengths of the intervention were found to be its promptness to complete research, to publish outputs and to showcase clinical innovations. The main barriers identified were time available to do research, appropriate support from academics and from peers. In terms of longer-term impacts, the majority of participants stated through the quantitative survey that they had increased experience at scientific writing and data analysis.

References

Banka Cullen, S., Lavelle, S., McDonagh, D., Walsh, R., & Comiskey, C. (2022). *In plain sight: A rapid review of the international Litera-ture and a National Estimate of the prevalence of women who use substances and experience domestic violence in Ireland*. S. Project. https://www.drugsandalcohol.ie/36282/1/DAVINA%20Report%20Final%20Revised%20May%202022.pdf

Burke, K., Morris, K., & McGarrigle, L. (2012). *An introductory guide to implementation: Terms, concepts and frameworks*. Centre for Effective Services.

CDC. (1999). *Framework for program evaluation in public health. MMWR 1999;48 (No. RR-11):1–42*. Centers for Disease Control and Prevention. Retrieved April 16, 2024 from https://www.cdc.gov/evaluation/materials/frameworksummary.pdf

CDC. (2021). *Evaluation steps*. Retrieved April 16, 2024 from https://www.cdc.gov/evaluation/steps/index.htm

Comiskey, C. M., O'Sullivan, K., Quirke, M. B., Wynne, C., Hollywood, E., & McGilloway, S. (2015). An analysis of the first implementation and impact of the World Health Organisation's health promoting school model within disadvantaged city schools in Ireland. *Vulnerable Children and Youth Studies, 10*(4), 281–293.

Comiskey, C. et al. (2018) An evaluation of the gay Men's health service outreach Programme, HSE Sexual Health & Crisis Pregnancy Programme. *ISBN 978-1-905199-44-0*. Available at: https://www.sexualwellbeing.ie/for-professionals/research/research-reports/gmhs-report_final.pdf. Accessed 03 June 2024.

Damschroder, L. J., Aron, D. C., Keith, R. E., Kirsh, S. R., Alexander, J. A., & Lowery, J. C. (2009). Fostering implementation of health services research findings into practice: a consolidated framework for advancing implementation science. *Implementation Science, 4*, 1–15.

Department of Health. (2018). *NCEC implementation guide and toolkit*. https://health.gov.ie/national-patient-safety-office/ncec/

Eccles, M. P., & Mittman, B. S. (2006). Welcome to implementation science. *Implementation Science, 1*(1), 1. https://doi.org/10.1186/1748-5908-1-1

EMCDDA. (2021). *Action framework for developing and implementing health and social responses to drug problems*. European Monitoring Centre for Drugs and Drug Addiction. Retrieved August 28, 2023 from https://www.emcdda.europa.eu/publications/mini-guides/action-framework-for-developing-and-implementing-health-and-social-responses-to-drug-problems_en#section2

Farrell, G., & Comiskey, C. (2014). Dualities of living with HIV/HCV co-infection: Patients' perspectives from those who are ineligible for or nonresponsive to treatment. *Journal of the Association of Nurses in AIDS Care, 25*(1), 9–22. https://doi.org/10.1016/j.jana.2012.10.005

Fixsen, D. L. (2005). *Implementation research: A synthesis of the literature*. National Implementation Research Network.

Glasgow, R. E., Vogt, T. M., & Boles, S. M. (1999). Evaluating the public health impact of health promotion interventions: The RE-AIM framework. *American Journal of Public Health, 89*(9), 1322–1327.

Gossop, M., Marsden, J., Stewart, D., & Rolfe, A. (2000). Patterns of improvement after methadone treatment: 1 year follow-up results from the National Treatment Outcome Research Study (NTORS). *Drug and Alcohol Dependence, 60*(3), 275–286.

IEG. (2024). *What is monitoring and evaluation?* . Independent Evaluation Group (IEG) of the World Bank Retrieved April 11, 2024 from https://ieg.worldbankgroup.org/what-monitoring-and-evaluation

Jobs, S. (1985, February 1). *Excerpt from an interview with David Sheff*, www.scribd.com. https://allaboutstevejobs.com/verbatim/interviews/playboy_1985

Kusek, J. Z., & Rist, R. C. (2004). *Ten steps to a results-based monitoring and evaluation system: a handbook for development practitioners*. World Bank Publications.

McGilloway, S., Bywater, T., Ni Mhaille, G., Furlong, M., O'Neill, D., Comiskey, C., Leckey, Y., Kelly, P., & Donnelly, M. , (2009). *Proving the power of positive parenting: A randomised controlled trial to investigate the effectiveness of the incredible years BASIC parenting training programme in an Irish context (short-term outcomes)*. I. Dublin, Archways. https://www.atlanticphilanthropies.org/wp-content/uploads/2015/09/Incredible-Years-Ireland-Study-Proving-the-Power-of-Positive-Parenting-Report.pdf

McKee, G., Codd, M., Dempsey, O., Gallagher, P., & Comiskey, C. (2017). Describing the implementation of an innovative intervention and evaluating its effectiveness in increasing research capacity of advanced clinical nurses: Using the consolidated framework for implementation research. *BMC Nursing, 16*, 1–13.

Metz, A., & Louison, L. (2019). The hexagon: An exploration tool. Hexagon discussion & analysis tool instructions. *National Implementation Research Network, Frank Porter Graham Child Development Institute, University of North Carolina at Chapel Hill. Based on Kiser, Zabel, Zachik, & Smith (2007) and Blase, Kiser & Van Dyke (2013)*. https://nirn.fpg.unc.edu/sites/nirn.fpg.unc.edu/files/imce/documents/NIRN%20Hexagon%20Discussion%20Analysis%20Tool%20v2.2.pdf

Metz, A., Naoom, S. F., Halle, T., & Bartley, L. (2015). *An integrated stage-based framework for implementation of early childhood programs and systems* (OPRE Research Brief OPRE 2015–48). Office of Planning. Research and Evaluation, Administration for Children and

Families, US Department of Health and Human Services. Retrieved April 10, 2024, from https://nirn.fpg.unc.edu/sites/nirn.fpg.unc.edu/files/resources/OPRE-stage_based_framework_brief_508.pdf

Moullin, J. C., Sabater-Hernández, D., Fernandez-Llimos, F., & Benrimoj, S. I. (2015). A systematic review of implementation frameworks of innovations in healthcare and resulting generic implementation framework. *Health Research Policy and Systems, 13*, 1–11.

Nickitas, D. M., & Feeg, V. (2011). Doubling the number of nurses with a doctorate by 2020: Predicting the right number or getting it right? *Nursing Economics, 29*(3), 109–112.

NIH. (2023). *Toolkit part 1: Implementation science methodologies and frameworks.* Fogarty International Centre, National Institute of Health. Retrieved April 11, 2024 from https://www.fic.nih.gov/About/center-global-health-studies/neuroscience-implementation-toolkit/Pages/methodologies-frameworks.aspx

Nilsen, P. (2020). Making sense of implementation theories, models, and frameworks. *Implementation Science, 3(0)*, 53–79.

Organization for Economic Co-operation and Development (OECD). (2023). Our global reach. Retrieved April 15, 2024 from https://www.oecd.org/about/members-and-partners/

RE-AIM. (2024). *RE-AIM*. Retrieved April 11, 2024 from https://re-aim.org/

Sheehan, A. M., While, A. E., & Coyne, I. (2015). The experiences and impact of transition from child to adult healthcare services for young people with type 1 diabetes: a systematic review. *Diabetic Medicine, 32*(4), 440–458. https://doi.org/10.1111/dme.12639

Simpson, D. D., Patrick, F. M., Joe, G., & Lehman, W. (2009). *Organizational readiness for change*. Texas Christian University. Institute of Behavioral Research. Retrieved April 11, 2024 from https://www.drugsandalcohol.ie/17872/

Smit, B., Williamson, C., & Padayachee, A. (2013). PhD capacity-building, from aid to innovation: The SANPAD-SANTRUST experience. *Studies in Higher Education, 38*(3), 441–455.

Wade, M. J. (2016). From Ockham's razor to rube Goldberg: Don't rely on forensic age-dating miracles. *Environmental Forensics, 17*(2), 131–135.

Wang, Y., Wong, E. L.-Y., Nilsen, P., Chung, V. C.-H., Tian, Y., & Yeoh, E.-K. (2023). A scoping review of implementation science theories, models, and frameworks—An appraisal of purpose, characteristics, usability, applicability, and testability. *Implementation Science, 18*(1), 43. https://doi.org/10.1186/s13012-023-01296-x

Chapter 11
Disruptive Innovation, Sustainability, and Sharing Best Practice: How to Be Innovative, Sustainable, and Share Learning

Setting the Scene

> *"I believe innovation is the most powerful force for change in the world." "As we look ahead into the next century, leaders will be those that empower others."* Bill Gates (Gates, 2024a, b)

> *eHealth interventions to combat addictive behaviours are burgeoning. There is an urgent need to take a more systematic approach to describing the content of these interventions and features of their delivery so that we can start to see patterns in what works for whom with what behaviours in what context.* John Cunningham (Cunningham, 2016, p. 389)

> *Countries must assess the implications of their drug policies for all relevant sections of their national plans to achieve the Sustainable Development Goals. They should determine the impact of drug policies on people's lives, on public safety and on the well-being of communities, as well as on social cohesion and development, as an integral part of measuring progress on the implementation of the 2030 Agenda for Sustainable Development.* (Global Commission on Drug Policy, 2018)

Introduction

From Bill Gates to Addiction editorials to the Global Commission on Drug Policy, the need for constant innovation, sustainable services and the sharing of learning has been hailed as essential tenets for the future of substance use policy, practice, and the provision of care. The Global Commission on Drug Policy has been calling for a paradigm shift. They wish to ensure that drug policies are reflecting the 17 Sustainable Development Goals (SDGs) and that services and practices promoted by those polices are underpinned by the six essential elements of the SDGs. These are justice-based, people-centered, dignity-orientated, solidarity-based partnerships that are respectful of the planet and focus on prosperity for all. Healthcare innovation and the sharing of best practice can contribute to these six elements and values.

C. Comiskey, *Addiction Research and Evaluation*, Advances in Mental Health and Addiction, https://doi.org/10.1007/978-3-031-65917-1_11

The World Health Organization's strategy for digital health (WHO, 2021) is to promote healthy lives and well-being for everyone, everywhere at all ages. To deliver this vision globally but also locally within policies, practices and services, national and local services must also develop their strategy focusing on the integration of financial, organizational, human, and technological resources. In support of their strategy (WHO, 2023) issued a global call to governments for action. They recognize that digital technologies are now a part of most people's everyday life, and that the world hasn't never been so interconnected.

Globally, innovation and digital health are expanding at a rapid rate. However, despite this growth the potential of digital health technologies to improve the lives of people who use substances, their families, and communities remains largely untapped. The WHO calls for a coordinated approach in health products and systems innovation to expand their use in low- and middle-income countries and to harness the power of these technologies to accelerate health and well-being and reduce disparities. In the words of the WHO:

> *This global Call to Action is intended to inspire governments and their innovation ecosystem partners worldwide to work together to accelerate the achievement of the Sustainable Development Goals (SDGs) through health innovation.*
>
> *We invite governments, international organizations, academia, industry leaders, and civil society to use it proactively in discussions among each other and with other governments and partners on how to use innovation, at scale, for the public good.* (WHO, 2023).

Within this chapter we explore the current hot topics in healthcare innovation and their possibilities for use in substance use services. We explore developing sustainable services and practice and finally we will provide guidance on sharing best practice. Case studies will illustrate in a practical way how some of these topics have been used at a local level.

Innovation

According to Marr (2023) published in *Forbes* magazine, longer living populations, transformative health technologies and their applications, along with global economic uncertainty, will be the drivers impacting healthcare in the near future. The transformative and disruptive nature of Artificial Intelligence (AI) will bring about great changes in how both health and care are delivered by services and received by people. According to Marr (2023) the top ten trends will be as outlined in Table 11.1.

Other authors agree broadly with Marr (2023). Nava (2023) puts forward her eight top developments and includes similar items, she is more specific in detailing Electronic Health Records and Robotics. Within her top eight. The World Economic Forum (Ellerbeck, 2023) in their listing of five innovations that are revolutionizing global healthcare also include AI, 3D printing, gene editing, VR, and finally smart bandages. These are bandages that use sensors to monitor and improve wound healing.

Table 11.1 The top ten trends in healthcare innovation according to *Forbes* business magazine (Marr, 2023)

	Innovation	Explanation and illustration
1.	Generative AI in healthcare	AI itself will be instrumental in many trends but generative AI which can learn from existing data to generate new data can be used to interpret results and generate personalized recommendations. It can create chatbots and virtual assistants to help at every stage of the patient journey. The applications of AI in healthcare are almost limitless
2.	Personalized (precision) medicine	This refers to the development of highly individualized treatment plans using technology and data. Currently the most advanced areas are in genomics where AI is being used to analyze a person's DNA. It is anticipated this will lead to better outcomes, increase efficiency and use of resources
3.	Virtual healthcare assistants	Virtual healthcare assistants and chatbots can assist both healthcare professionals and patients by providing advice on treatments and medications. They can connect patients with information they may need to make decisions, remind them to take their medications and also provide some companionship
4.	Digital twinning (of an object, system or process)	A digital twin is a virtual model of a real world item. It can be used to simulate the actual item or system and explore the impact of modifications. Digital twins of human organs have been developed to model the effects of changes in treatment etc.
5.	Internet of things (IoT) powered virtual hospitals and telemedicine 2.0	This includes both telemedicine and wearable devices connected to the global network known as the Internet of things (IoT). The term telemedicine 2.0 is used as it goes beyond simple online consultations to include more holistic care. As the growth in remote monitoring expands there is potential for virtual hospital wards, where a central location acts as a hub for monitoring patients in their own homes, again reducing resources needed
6.	Preventative healthcare	A global shift from healthcare providers to an emphasis on prevention rather than cure, is emerging as it is beneficial for people and reduces costs for providers. Technological advances including AI and wearable technology will have a key role in prevention as these technologies can provide early warning signs and rapid interventions
7.	Virtual reality and augmented reality	Virtual reality (VR) which is an immersive experience has been used to assist with pain management in cancer treatments. One example is the transporting of patients to other inspiring locations while they received their chemotherapy. Augmented reality (AR) unlike VR is within a real-world setting but with additional information. It can provide healthcare professionals with additional information without having to look at screens
8.	Elderly care	As many countries encounter ageing populations who are living longer, innovative solutions to enable people to stay in their homes longer and new treatments for conditions that occur in older age are being developed
9.	3D printing	3D printing of implants, tools, and devices is growing. This has the potential to have a major impact on healthcare in regions where healthcare equipment is scare. It has been used to print surgical instruments, orthopedic and dental implants and prosthetics

(continued)

Table 11.1 (continued)

	Innovation	Explanation and illustration
10.	Convergence of mental and physical healthcare delivery	To date, the delivery of physical and mental health services has been separated each operating within their own silo with patients travelling from one service to another. Marr (2023) within this selection of the top ten innovations of the near future highlights that since the COVID-19 pandemic we have all learned that these are inseparable. Frontline staff in the near future will be increasingly addressing both in the pursuit of overall well-being

Finally in an analysis of over 3600 start-up companies (StartUs Insights, 2024) in their top ten trends include big data and analytics, cloud computing, and blockchain technology. Blockchain technology enables the decentralization of a ledger of data that stores the records of ownership of any digital assets. Data stored on blockchain cannot be modified and is therefore protected. It enables secure transactions and apart from its original use in moving money it is emerging as a means of safeguarding healthcare records, remote patient monitoring, pharmaceutical supply chains, and health insurance claims.

Clearly there are global innovations being developed at an increasing rate, the question is, how are addiction services taking advantage of these developments?

Definitions of eHealth, mHealth, and Digital Health Within Substance Use

WHO defines eHealth as, the cost-effective and secure use of information and communications technologies in support of health and health-related fields, including health-care services, health surveillance, health literature, and health education, knowledge and research (WHO, 2021). To explore the use of these innovations in addressing drug use the European Monitoring Centre for Drugs and Drug Addiction (EMCDDA) commissioned a background paper on this topic by Blankers and Mujcic (2017). According to Blankers and Mujcic (2017), the use of digital (computer-based) technologies for health is referred to as eHealth. Examples of regular practices supported by eHealth within substance use are the treatment of clients via Internet or computer-based interventions, education of professions working in addiction services via eLearning courses and client monitoring via wearable technology or digitalized diaries.

Mobile digital technologies to support practices are referred to as mHealth, as an abbreviation of mobile health. This involves services and programs accessed thorough wireless networks and mobile devices such as smart phones. mHealth is one part of eHealth. The term digital health according to WHO was introduced as a term to include eHealth (which includes mHealth) and the burgeoning fields, of advanced computing sciences in "big data," genomics and artificial intelligence.

A spotlight summarizing eHealth and mHealth was developed by the EMCDDA (2023) for substance use services. The spotlight notes three main groups of mHealth, mobile phone applications. These are detailed in Fig. 11.1.

Capacity building for professionals is part of a key priority for the Substance Abuse and Mental Health Services Administration strategic plan 2023–2026 within the United States (SAMHSA, 2023). Within their priority 5 area of strengthening the workforce, they seek to increase accessibility of service providers to those in need by expanding virtual services and increase training for staff in this area. This focus on staff development is also expressed by the WHO (2021) in their global strategy on digital health where they highlight the importance of integrating financial, organization, technological, and human resources.

What Digital Intervention Works for Whom and Where?

Johansson et al. (2024) in their systematic review of digital interventions targeting substance use (alcohol, tobacco, and other drugs) from 2015 to 2022 mapped the literature to identify neglected and emerging knowledge gaps. They reviewed over 3000 studies including other reviews and meta-analyses. They also reported on any theoretical foundations within the interventions and found that two thirds of the papers provided these details. This is an important point for future intervention adoption or development. From the meta-analyses of several Cochrane reviews on different substances they found that digital interventions had significant effects and that longer interventions were more effective than shorter ones.

Looking at the effects of different technologies, they found that text messaging for smoking cessation was effective as an adjunct to other interventions. Smoking cessation apps showed no effects compared with minimal interventions. However, they also found that digital smoking cessation resulted in higher smoking abstinence, when delivered via web, as well as via mobile or via text messages when

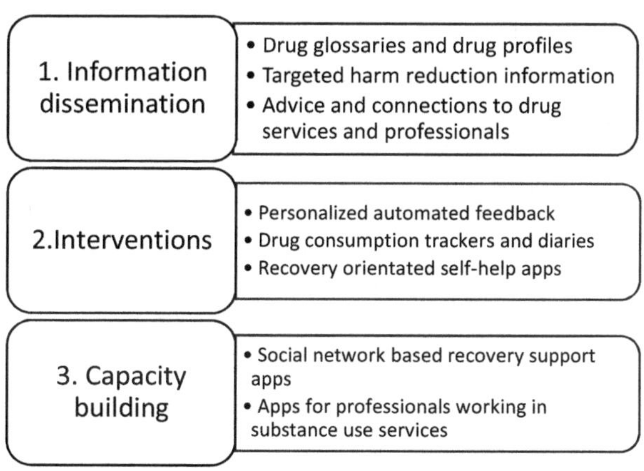

Fig. 11.1 Three common topics that can be addressed by mHealth applications for substance use. (Adapted from EMCDDA, 2023)

compared to inactive control groups. From these findings it is clear that prior to introducing a digital intervention for smoking cessation a detailed review of the smoking findings of Johansson et al. (2024) would be prudent.

In terms of alcohol and other drugs the effects of mobile and text interventions to reduce the use of these substances was unclear. A review of mobile apps showed that although most people reduced their use, less than a third of studies showed significantly better effects compared to comparisons. With regards to text message interventions, one meta-analysis found that it was unclear whether they reduced weekly consumption. A key finding was that few of the most common app for substance use had scientific support or used evidence-based methods. This is another important factor to consider if adopting or developing a digital intervention. Wearable sensors and other wireless technology can be used to monitor substance use or reduce the risk of overdose or relapse, but the effects of such interventions are still unclear.

Exploring theoretical groundings, digital cognitive behavior for alcohol use was found to be effective in comparison with minimal control interventions and as an adjunct to usual treatment. A review of motivational interviewing (MI) to reduce substance use found that MI via telephone was effective and that positive effects for text and Internet-based MI have been observed in a smaller number of studies, for alcohol.

Johansson et al. (2024) also reviewed specific population groups and settings. These included school settings, young people, students, older people, and women. It was found that digital universal prevention primarily delivered in schools found significant but moderately-sized effects on alcohol or drug use outcomes of six youth programs. A meta-analysis of digital interventions in school that targeted changes in several health behaviors simultaneously showed no effects on alcohol or tobacco. If designing school-based interventions, it would appear that a narrower focusing of the intervention is important.

One further key finding was that many studies have not assessed gender-specific effects and that support for specific effects among women with substance use problems is therefore weak and this needs to be addressed. Table 11.2 provides a summary of some key messages from this comprehensive review of digital interventions.

Table 11.2 A summary of six key learnings on the efficacy of digital interventions. (Based on Johansson et al., 2024)

1.	A theoretical foundation and scientific evidence for a digital intervention is important
2.	Longer interventions are more effective than shorter ones
3.	Digital interventions as an adjunct to an existing intervention can be more effective
4.	Cognitive behavioral therapy and motivational interviewing as a grounding in a digital intervention can be effective with some substances
5.	Focused school-based interventions targeting specific substances as opposed to more broad-based interventions can be effective
6.	Evidence of gender-specific effects are weak and more focus on results for women should be included

Substance Use Services and Addressing the Sustainable Development Goals

The Global Commission on Drug Policy (2018) has been calling for a paradigm shift in international, national, and local drug policies. They believe that drug policies should be underpinned by six essential elements of the SDGs. These being, justice-based, people-orientated, dignity-orientated, solidarity-based partnerships that are respectful of the planet and focus on prosperity for all. They believe that the 17 sustainable development goals in Fig. 11.2 are meant to be transformative in eradicating poverty, gender inequity and protect the planet through their implementation. The challenges of poverty, gender inequity, lack of access to education, and health services are more pronounced among people who use substances and the famers and workers who are involved in their production. A policy briefing to the UNODC from Health Poverty Action (2015) provides an excellent summary of this and of how drug policy and service reform is essential to achieving aspects of each of the SDGs.

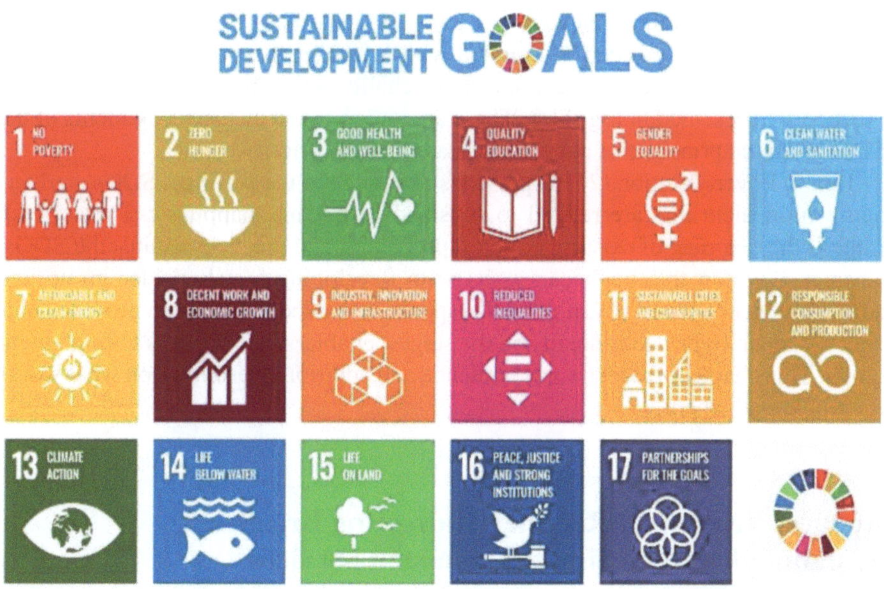
SUSTAINABLE DEVELOPMENT GOALS
1 NO POVERTY
2 ZERO HUNGER
3 GOOD HEALTH AND WELL-BEING
4 QUALITY EDUCATION
5 GENDER EQUALITY
6 CLEAN WATER AND SANITATION
7
8 DECENT WORK AND ECONOMIC GROWTH
9 INDUSTRY, INNOVATION AND INFRASTRUCTURE
10 REDUCED INEQUALITIES
11
12 RESPONSIBLE CONSUMPTION AND PRODUCTION
13 CLIMATE ACTION
14 LIFE BELOW WATER
15 LIFE ON LAND
16 PEACE, JUSTICE AND STRONG INSTITUTIONS
17 PARTNERSHIPS FOR THE GOALS

Fig. 11.2 The 17 sustainable development goals with further details available from (https://www.un.org/sustainabledevelopment) (Available to download at https://www.un.org/sustainabledevelopment/news/communications-material/ Please note that the content of this publication has not been approved by the United Nations and does not reflect the views of the United Nations or its officials or Member States.)

Defining Sustainability of Innovation in Policy or Practice

According to the Department of Health (2018, p. 42), the United Kingdom's National Health Service (NHS, 2005, p. 18) defines sustainability within healthcare as being achieved not only when process and outcomes have changed but also the thinking and attitudes behind them are fundamentally altered and the systems around them are transformed as well. The change has become an integrated or mainstream way of working rather than something added on. The Department of Health (2018) when speaking of sustaining change after an intervention, state that a change has been sustained if 1 year or longer at a minimum, the situation has not reverted to the previous ways of working. The same criteria for defining sustainability within innovations can be made when implementing new innovations into services.

Six Stages to Achieving Sustainable Innovation in Addiction Policy and Practice

The WHO (2023), within their innovation hub state that they "*use sustainable innovation to solve bottlenecks, accelerate impact and improve health, focusing on the most neglected problems and people*." People who use drugs and alcohol are included under this remit. They provide a five-staged process for addressing sustainable innovation and this can be coupled with learnings from other chapters within this book. An adaptation of these stages for challenges within addiction policy and practice are presented in Fig. 11.3. These are underpinned by the six elements of the SDGs with the principle of people-orientated taking priority.

Health Poverty Action (2015) provides examples of the pertinent SDGs, and targets within them that are related to substance use. This mapping can assist with stage 1, the mapping of existing policies, processes, and practices against the SDGs. Chapter 3 within this book can assist with developing a stakeholder group and addressing needs. Similarly, if a rapid response is needed Chap. 6 can provide guidance. Chapter 10 provides details on the stages, enablers, and barriers to implementation. This chapter provides some evidence and additional resources on what works for whom and where.

Reduce, Reuse, and Recycle: Addressing Broader Sustainability and Climate Change in Services

The impact of climate change on health is well established from the impacts of heat wave-related impacts to the rise in flood and storm-related impacts. Related to these there are global rises in respiratory diseases and in waterborne diseases (HSE, 2023). National governments are increasingly aware of the need to address this

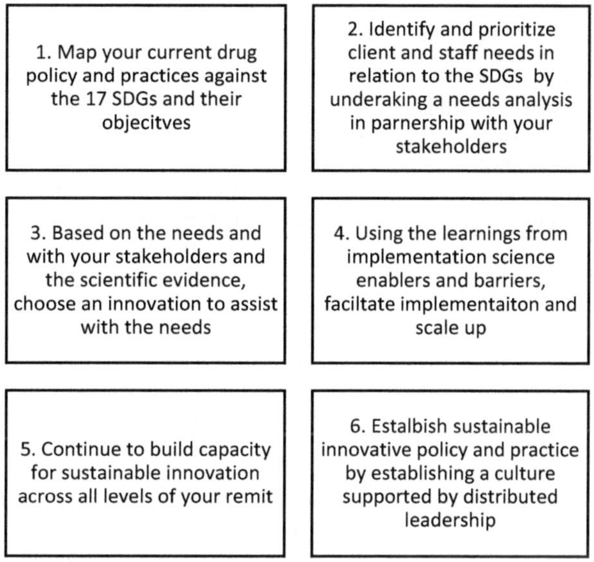

Fig. 11.3 A six-staged framework to achieving sustainable innovation in addiction policy and practice

within all aspects of their ministries. One ministry within Ireland have produced a climate strategy with a vision to achieve net-zero emissions by 2050. They provide some guidance for services and details on things that can be accomplished now to help (HSE, 2024).

A summary of areas where leadership and staff can integrate sustainable practices is provided in Table 11.3. The integration of sustainable practices is an example of where distributed leadership discussed in Chap. 9 can have a significant impact.

Identifying Best Practice

At the opening of this chapter, Bill Gates was quoted as saying *"leaders will be those that empower others,"* (Gates, 2024b). If others are to be empowered then sharing of learning and particularly the sharing of best practice needs to occur not just within and from research institutions but from practice and peers.

How can best practice be identified, shared, and disseminated? WHO (2008) provides a detailed guide for documenting and sharing best practice. Within this they also provide a definition and guidance on recognizing best practice. They define best practice as meeting the criteria of effectiveness, efficiency and relevance in addition to one or more of the other criteria. Best practice need not meet all of the criteria. These criteria for selecting best practice within substance use services are detailed in Table 11.4.

Table 11.3 Areas within addiction services where sustainability can be addressed. (Adapted from HSE (2024), where additional simple suggestions for change can be found)

Area to be addressed	Some suggested approaches within addiction services
Sustainable buildings and service environment	This might include both the internal and external building environment where your service is delivered. For example, do you have a green space for staff and clients?
Transport and mobility	Are clients asked to travel to treatment centers more often than is necessary? Can they take home medications or can they get order and receive their prescriptions online using mHealth?
Sustainable procurement	Can a current product you are purchasing be changed from a disposable product to a reusable one? Can you ask your supplier to use recycled packaging?
Greener models of healthcare	Can you avail of more online meetings and consultations to avoid unnecessary travel? Can you develop satellite services where a few staff travel to a location instead of many clients travelling to your service?
Water and waste management	Can you fit your water supply taps with water savers to reduce flow? Can you fix leaking taps? To reduce waste can you go plastic free? Do you provide well-labeled garbage bins for waste to be appropriately recycled?
Adaption and developing resilience	Is your service proactive and consultative in addressing staff and client concerns for the future? Do you have a sustainability working group?

Table 11.4 Criteria for assessing what is best practice within substance use services. (Adapted from WHO, 2008)

Key criteria
1. Effectiveness, the practice has been demonstrated to work in a meaningful and measurable way
2. Efficiency, the practice produces results within reasonable resource usage
3. Relevance, the practice addresses a priority for addiction services practitioners or clients
Plus at least one of the additional criteria
4. Ethical, the practice reflects internationally accepted ethical standards
5. Sustainable, the practice reaches the definition of sustainable as articulated within this chapter
6. Duplicable, the practice is capable of being replicated within other addiction services
7. Involves partnerships, the practice involves appropriate non-tokenistic partnerships with stakeholders
8. Community involvement, the practice involves participation of the communities affected
9. Political commitment, the practice has the support of the relevant local, regional or national authorities

Sharing Learning

In terms of generating learning for best practice and the sharing of that learning, stakeholder engagement is a key component. Models for citizens participation and meaningful engagement were first proposed by Arnstein in the 1960s. Arnstein (1969) defines citizen participation as, "*the strategy by which the have nots join in determining how information is shared, goals and policies are set, tax resources are allocated, programs are operated, and benefits like contracts and patronage are parcelled out.*" She presents a typology of eight levels of participation to help address the confusion and lack of understanding on this topic. Her eight levels are represented in a hierarchy on a ladder, and these have formed the foundations for many stakeholder engagement strategies.

In summary the levels fall into three categories, nonparticipation, degrees of tokenism and degrees of power. Within nonparticipation the first two rungs of the ladder are manipulation and therapy, where the objective is to "educate" and "cure" participants. Rungs 3 and 4 are informing and consultation, where power holders provide opportunities to hear and be heard but where participants are not heeded. Rung 5 is simple placation, where power holders allow the have-nots to advise but not decide. Rung 6 is partnership which allows for negotiation and trade off, rung 7 is delegated power, and rung 8 is citizen control.

An example of citizen control might be a neighborhood collective being allocated an addiction service budget and having control over how that budget was spent. To achieve shared learning a partnership approach at least is needed if the criteria of relevance, effectiveness, and efficiency are to be met when the service or practice is implemented with all stakeholders.

Measuring the Impact of a Best Practice

The European Union through its Horizon Program (Horizon Europe, 2023) along with many other international and national funders have made the measurement of impact an essential component of funding granted for research. The day of ivory towers where research was for the elite have long passed and it is the responsibility of those who receive funding, be it for research or for service development and delivery, to demonstrate how they are making a difference. To assist with this Horizon Europe (2023) have identified key impact pathways that with adaption, addiction policies, services, and practices can use to measure the breath of their work's impact beyond the usual monitoring and evaluation. This is summarized in Table 11.5.

Dissemination

In terms of a dissemination strategy of the shared learning and best practice developed, Nottingham Trent University in the United Kingdom provide a nice toolkit to assist with this (NTU, 2024). They highlight that an effective dissemination strategy relies on the use of various media and audiences. They provide a series of questions within their toolkit to help direct and focus your dissemination. This includes questions about the aim and objective of your dissemination strategy, your audience who will benefit, the mediums you will use to disseminate and finally a template to assist

Table 11.5 Key impact pathways for addiction research, policy, practice, and services

Scientific impact	Creating high-quality new knowledge for addiction research, policy, practice, and service
	Strengthening human capital in research and innovation among addiction professionals and the people they work with
	Fostering diffusion of knowledge and open source sharing of learning across all stakeholders
Societal impact	Addressing EU policy priorities and global challenges in addiction through research and innovation
	Delivering benefits and impact within addiction and addiction related services and people through research and innovation missions
	Strengthening the uptake of research and innovation in addiction policy, practice, and services
Technological and economic impact	Generating innovation-based growth in addiction policy, practice, and services
	Creating more and better jobs
	Leveraging investment in research and innovation for the betterment of addiction policy, practice, services, and the staff and stakeholders who engage with them

Adapted from Horizon Europe (2023), program analysis

with your dissemination. As most dissemination strategies will involve the use of social media there are also guides on keeping the message professional. A simple guide is produced by the Nursing and Midwifery Board of Ireland (2013). They have summarized the guide into the six P's. These are, keep it professional; keep posts positive; keep posts person or patient free; protect your professionalism; check your privacy settings; and finally pause before you post.

Best Practice Guidelines and Portals

Many international organizations provide access to best practice guidelines and information on addiction-related interventions and programs. These can be freely accessed to guide your policy, practice, or service. Similarly, a program or intervention can be submitted to these organizations for an external validation and possible inclusion within their portals. A small and diverse sample is provided in Table 11.6 with a brief explanation. In addition, globally the World Health Organization together and United Nations Office on Drugs and Crime (2020) have produced an international standards document for the treatment of drug use disorders.

To conclude this chapter, two case studies are provided below illustrating some of the learnings highlighted and applied in practice.

Case Study 11.1: Developing Staff Capacity and Sharing Learning with an Innovative and Free MOOC (Massive Open Online Course)

Introduction

Nurses and midwives working across city center addiction services wished to improve their practice from one that was reactive to one that was proactive. They wished to address their caseloads which were defined as all clients registered with the network of services across the city. This included opiate agonist treatment services, infectious disease clinics, maternity clinics for women who were pregnant and used substances and satellite community clinics for people who use drugs and were living on the outskirts of the city. Working with an academic team; international evidence on best practice in nursing models; clients who use substances and staff, they developed an addiction nursing model and a manual to describe how to implement it. This model had the client at the center, was cognizant of the setting, used brief intervention approaches and was measurable in terms of outcomes. Details are available at Comiskey et al. (2018); Comiskey et al. (2019); Comiskey et al. (2021); and Flanagan (2022).

Methods

The nurses and midwives wished to share their learning beyond their immediate colleagues. Continuing to work with stakeholders and the academic team they sought additional funding from their nursing and midwifery programming development unit. Funding was granted for the development of a Massive Open Online Course or MOOC. These are internationally open and free courses that can be accessed globally.

The aims of the MOOC were to provide additional training for nurses, midwives, and allied healthcare professionals working with people who use substances including:

- Best practice in assessment and screening, brief intervention, and overdose.
- Key addiction-related topics from maternity services through to older age.
- Trauma & Adverse Childhood Events.
- Guidance on leadership and implementation of the Healthy Addiction Treatment (HAT) model in practice.

Working with an international professional MOOC development company who host the online MOOCS, the team began the task. The steps involved in the MOOC are outlined in Fig. 11.4 and each of these was created by the team. The videos involved the creation of short scripts by the team and were based on real-life scenarios which had occurred in practice. They also involved the recruitment of

Table 11.6 A sample of best practice portals and guidelines for drug and alcohol services

African Union	African Union Compendium of Best Practices Published in 2020, this work showcases best practices in addressing drug use challenges in Africa. The articles in the publication were compiled and submitted by AU Member States Drug Demand Reduction National Focal points. The compendium was produced with an aim of sharing knowledge and enabling countries in Africa to benefit from sharing experiences and solutions on what works and draw on lessons learnt. Available at https://au.int/en/documents/20201030/compendium-good-practices-drug-use-prevention-drug-use-disorders-treatment-and Accessed April 26th 2024.
Australia	National Framework for Alcohol, Tobacco and Other Drug Treatment 2019–29 This framework's aim is to provide all Australians seeking alcohol and other drug treatment with access to quality treatment appropriate to their needs, when and where they need it. It includes details for effective treatment, monitoring and evaluation. Available at https://www.health.gov.au/resources/publications/national-framework-for-alcohol-tobacco-and-other-drug-treatment-2019-29?language=en Accessed April 26th 2024.
Canada	Registered Nurses Association Ontario (RNAO) Guidelines The RNAO have established a repository of over 50 best practice guidelines covering to date nine categories including mental health and substance use. Available at https://rnao.ca/bpg/guidelines Accessed April 26th, 2024.
Europe	The European Commission's Best Practice Portal This portal is designed to help find reliable and practical information on implemented practices recognized as best or promising in the area of public health. It includes communicable diseases such as HIV/AIDS, tuberculosis and viral hepatitis. Practices can be submitted for evaluation through this Best Practice Portal. Available at https://webgate.ec.europa.eu/dyna/bp-portal/ Accessed April 26th, 2024.
Europe	The European Monitoring Centre for Drugs and Drug Addiction (EMCDDA) Best Practice Portal This portal is designed to help one find practical and reliable information on what works in the areas of prevention, treatment, harm reduction and social reintegration. It helps to quickly identify tested interventions to ensure that resources are allocated to only those that are effective. Available at https://www.emcdda.europa.eu/best-practice_en Accessed April 26th, 2024.
Southeast Asia	The United Nations Office for Drugs and Crime (UNODC) have produced a guidance document Guidance for Community-Based Treatment and Care Services for People Affected by Drug Use and Dependence in Southeast Asia. At the time of publication, the dominant response in Southeast Asia to drug use and dependence was compulsory centers for people who use drugs. This Guidance Document outlines community-based treatment as an alternative model to compulsory centers. It is aimed at helping practitioners in the health, social work and law enforcement sectors implement community-based treatment. Available at https://www.unodc.org/documents/drug-treatment/UNODC_cbtx_guidance_EN.pdf Accessed 26th, 2024.

(continued)

Table 11.6 (continued)

United Kingdom	National Institute of Clinical Excellence (NICE) Guidelines This contains evidence-based recommendations for the health and social care sector, developed by independent committees, including professionals and lay members, and consulted on by stakeholders. Available at https://www.nice.org.uk/guidance Accessed 26th, 2024.
United States of America	Substance Abuse and Mental Health Services Administration (SAMHSA) SAMHSA aims to improve prevention, treatment, and recovery support services for mental and substance use disorders. Their Evidence-Based Practices Resource Center provides communities, clinicians, policymakers and others with the information and tools to incorporate evidence-based practices into their communities or clinical settings. Available at https://www.samhsa.gov/resource-search/ebp Accessed 26th, 2024.

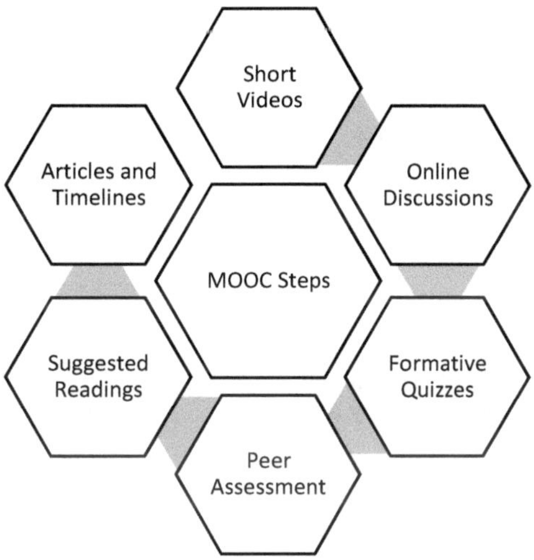

Fig. 11.4 The steps involved in an addiction MOOC development and resulting types of content experienced by participants in their training

professional actors and filmmakers. The MOOC development company provided access to these services.

Results

The final MOOC design consisted of the 6 h of content delivered over 3 weeks for participants. The details of the weekly topics and related materials are provided in Table 11.7.

Approximately 3000 people have engaged with the MOOC. Feedback has been positive, as can be seen in the selection of participant quotes provided in Fig. 11.5.

Discussion

The development of this innovative MOOC was shared across international academics, practitioners, clients, and experts in MOOC development. The combination of stakeholders resulted in a well-received product which has been shared across numerous countries and professionals. It remains available to all and can be accessed at https://www.futurelearn.com/courses/identifying-and-responding-to-drug-and-alcohol-addiction (Accessed April 26th 2024.)

Table 11.7 Topics covered in the 6 h of materials provided within the addiction MOOC

Weekly topics, weeks 1 to 3	Weekly materials to be covered in 2 h
Week 1: Treatment approaches & the individual Risk & protective factors Assessment & screening for substance abuse Supporting users via brief interventions Administering naloxone	Background academic information Short film with actors on conducting a drug & alcohol assessment using a trauma-informed approach Short film with actors on providing a brief intervention for a service user with anxiety & substance use, using a trauma-informed approach Tool kits for working with people with problematic substance use Real-life voices from service users about their experience of overdose Community key worker's experience of administering naloxone
Week 2: Trauma-informed care, the family & related challenges Trauma-informed service Adverse childhood events Women & pregnancy Ageing & substance abuse Infectious disease & increased risk Blood-borne viruses	Academic background information Interview with Dublin-based drug liaison midwife specialist: Pregnancy & substance use South African experience—discussion about needs of pregnant women with violent experiences Ethiopian experience—community perspective of risks for women with drug use Voices of service users about age-based experiences at entry to drug support services Discussion with two addiction service nurses regarding specific challenges of early & late onset addiction Discussion with Hepatitis C liaison nurse specialist: Examples of trauma-informed practice when diagnosing & treating Hepatitis C
Week 3: Leadership & improving your practice Leadership & improving your practice Using models for practice Leading the way—distributed leadership Identifying client needs The Healthy Addiction Treatment Model (H.A.T.) Implementing change & case management	Academic background information Leadership interview with ADON about how H.A.T. was developed & implemented in Dublin North Addiction Service Service user voices reflecting on their experience of healthcare & suggestions for improvements to enhance engagement and holistic care

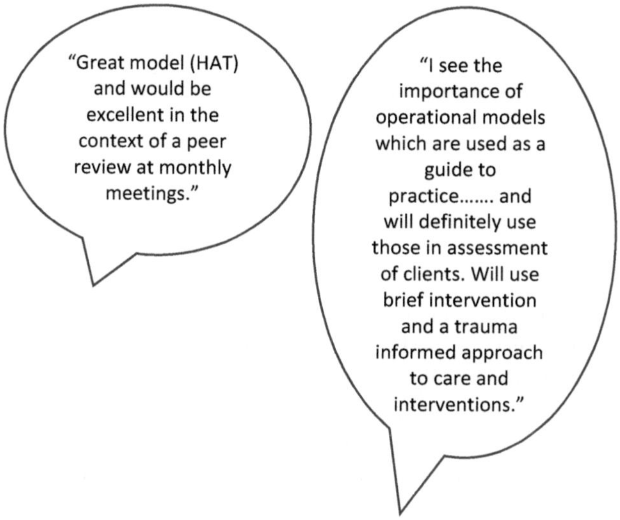

Fig. 11.5 Some feedback from participants undertaking the addiction MOOC

Case Study 11.2: Sample Cases from the World Health Organization Innovation Hub

Introduction

The Innovation Hub of the WHO (WHO, 2024) has the vision of a world in which everyone can live healthy, productive lives, regardless of who they are or where they live. They strive to support this vision using innovation.

Methods

The Hub collaborates with member states, the WHO workforce and external partners to improve and accelerate public health by leveraging innovative approaches to change. These approaches include a wide variety of innovations from the use of drones, to using containers to establish telehealth clinics in rural areas, to music therapy for mothers with mental health challenges and for people who experience drug addiction.

Results

The details and findings of just some of the innovations used are reported in detail (WHO, 2024).

Discussion

Many of the innovations described by the WHO could be adapted and be used for sustainable policies, services and practices with people who use drugs and alcohol. For example, in Somalia the WHO have harnessed solar power to deliver oxygen and electrify health facilities in remote and hard to reach locations. Similarly, telehealth addiction clinics could be established in rural areas using mHealth where community Internet infrastructure is not available but where smart phones are in use by individuals.

To conclude, this chapter recognizes that innovation is for all, not just those with access to expensive technology and services. Rather it is the responsibility of policy makers and practitioners to strive to bring these innovations to all so they may benefit all. In the words of Nelson Mandela,

> *Vision without action is just a dream, action without vision just passes the time, and vision with action can change the world.*
> *(Nelson Mandela, 1918–2013)*

References

Arnstein, S. R. (1969). A ladder of citizen participation. *Journal of the American Institute of Planners, 35*(4), 216–224. https://www.tandfonline.com/doi/abs/10.1080/01944366908977225

Blankers, M., & Mujcic, A. (2017). *E-health and m-health: Using new technologies to respond to drug problems.* European Monitoring Centre for Drugs and Drug Addiction Retrieved April 22, 2024 from https://www.emcdda.europa.eu/document-library/e-health-and-m-health-using-new-technologies-respond-drug-problems_en

Comiskey, C., Galligan, K., Banka, P., O'Brien Green, S., & McDonagh, D. (2018). *An evaluation of the gays men's health out-reach programme.* (ISBN 978-1-905199-44-0). Retrieved November 23, 2023, from https://www.sexualwellbeing.ie/for-professionals/research/research-reports/gmhs-report_final.pdf

Comiskey, C., Galligan, K., Flanagan, J., Deegan, J., Farnann, J., & Hall, A. (2019). Clients' views on the importance of a nurse-led approach and nurse prescribing in the development of the healthy addiction treatment recovery model. *Journal of Addictions Nursing, 30*(3), 169–176.

Comiskey, C., Galligan, K., Flanagan, J., Deegan, J., Farnann, J., & Hall, A. (2021). The healthy addiction treatment recovery model: Developing a client-driven, nurse-led addiction nursing model. *Journal of Addictions Nursing, 32*(1), E11–E20.

Cunningham, J. A. (2016). Addiction and eHealth. *Addiction, 111*(3), 389–390. https://doi.org/10.1111/add.13243

Department of Health. (2018). *NCEC implementation guide and Toolkit*. https://health.gov.ie/national-patient-safety-office/ncec/

Ellerbeck, S. (2023). *5 innovations that are revolutionizing global healthcare*. World Economnic Forum. Retrieved April 23, 2024 from https://www.weforum.org/agenda/2023/02/health-future-innovation-technology/

EMCDDA. (2023). *E-health and m-health: Using new technologies to respond to drug problems*. Retrieved April 25, 2024 from https://www.emcdda.europa.eu/document-library/e-health-and-m-health-using-new-technologies-respond-drug-problems_en

Flanagan, J. (2022). *Embedding a new model of care in addiction nursing: How one team's journey influenced behaviours & practices across wider frontiers*. Retrieved February 26, 2024 from https://healthservice.hse.ie/filelibrary/onmsd/embedding-a-new-model-of-care-in-addiction-nursing-jean-flanagan.pdf

Gates, B. (2024a). n.d.1. AZ Quotes.com. Retrieved April 22, 2024 from https://www.azquotes.com/quote/851057

Gates, B. (2024b). n.d.2. AZ Quotes.com. Retrieved April 22, 2024 from https://www.azquotes.com/quote/107324

Global Commission on Drug Policy. (2018). *Drug policy and the sustainable development Agenda*. Retrieved April 24, 2024 from https://www.globalcommissionondrugs.org/position-papers/sustainable-development-agenda-position-paper

Health Poverty Action. (2015). *Drug policy and the sustainable development goals*. Retrieved April 24, 2024 from https://www.unodc.org/documents/ungass2016/Contributions/Civil/Health_Poverty_Action/HPA_SDGs_drugs_policy_briefing_WEB.pdf

Horizon Europe. (2023). *Horizon Europe programme analysis: Impact assessment, evaluation and monitoring of Horizon Europe*. European Commission (europa.eu). https://research-and-innovation.ec.europa.eu/strategy/support-policy-making/shaping-eu-research-and-innovation-policy/evaluation-impact-assessment-and-monitoring/horizon-europe-programme-analysis_en

HSE. (2023). *HSE Climate Action Strategy 2023–2050*. https://www.hse.ie/eng/about/who/health-businessservices/national-health-sustainability-office/climate-change-and-health/hse-climate-action-strategy-2023-50.pdf

HSE. (2024). *Climate change and health*. Health Service The Executive Retrieved April 25, 2024 from.

Johansson, M., Romero, D., Jakobson, M., Heinemans, N., & Lindner, P. (2024). Digital interventions targeting excessive substance use and substance use disorders: A comprehensive and systematic scoping review and bibliometric analysis. *Frontiers in Psychiatry, 15*, 1233888.

Marr, B. (2023, October 3). The ten biggest trends revolutionizing healthcare in 2024. *Forbes Magazine*. Retrieved April 24, 2024 from https://www.forbes.com/sites/bernardmarr/2023/10/03/the-10-biggest-trends-revolutionizing-healthcare-in-2024/

Nava, C. (2023, March 21). How technology is changing the future of healthcare. *HealthTech*. Retrieved April 23, 2024 from https://www.healthtechzone.com/topics/healthcare/articles/2023/03/21/455345-how-technology-changing-future-healthcare.htm

NHS. (2005). *Sustainability: Model and guide*. NHS Institute for Innovation and Improvement.

NTU. (2024). *Dissemination strategy. What is your GAME plan?* . NTU Nottingham Trent University. Retrieved April 24, 2024 from NTU Nottingham Trent University (2024) Available at https://www.ntu.ac.uk/__data/assets/pdf_file/0028/865711/dissemination-game-plan.pdf

Nursing and Midwifery Board of Ireland. (2013). *Guidance to nurses and midwives on social media and social networking*. https://www.nmbi.ie/nmbi/media/NMBI/Publications/Guidance-to-Nurses-Midwives-on-Social-Media-Social-Networking.pdf?ext=.pdf.

SAMHSA. (2023). *Strategic Plan: Fiscal Year 2023–2026* (Publication No. PEP23-06-00-002 MD). https://www.samhsa.gov/homeless-housing-resource-center

StartUs Insights. (2024). *Explore the top 10 healthcare trends & innovations in 2024*. https://www.startus-insights.com/innovators-guide/top-10-healthcare-industry-trends-innovations-in-2021/#blockchain

WHO. (2008). *Guide for documenting and sharing best practice in health programmes*. World Health Organization. Retrieved April 25, 2024 from https://www.afro.who.int/sites/default/files/2017-06/Guide_for_documenting_and_Sharing_Best_Practice_-_english_0.pdf

WHO. (2021). *Global strategy on digital health 2020–2025. Licence: CC BY-NC-SA 3.0 IGO*. World Health Organization. https://www.who.int/publications/i/item/9789240020924

WHO. (2023). Global call to action for health innovation scale-up by the public sector. *Licence: CC BY-NC-SA 3.0 IGO*. World Health Organization. https://iris.who.int/bitstream/handle/10665/375598/9789240084698-eng.pdf?sequence=1&isAllowed=y

WHO. (2024). WHO innovation hub. World Health Organization. Retrieved April 26, 2024 from https://www.who.int/teams/digital-health-and-innovation/who-innovation-hub

World Health Organization and United Nations Office on Drugs and Crime. (2020) *International standards for the treatment of drug use disorders: Revised edition incorporating results of field-testing. License: CC BY-NC-SA 3.0 IGO*. Available at: https://www.unodc.org/documents/UNODC-WHO-Interational_Standards_Treatment_DrugUseDisorders_121217.pdf. Accessed 03 June 2024.

Index

C. Comiskey, *Addiction Research and Evaluation*, Advances in Mental Health and Addiction, https://doi.org/10.1007/978-3-031-65917-1

R

S

T

U

V

MIX
Papier aus verantwortungsvollen Quellen
Paper from responsible sources
FSC® C105338

If you have any concerns about our products,
you can contact us on
ProductSafety@springernature.com

In case Publisher is established outside the EU,
the EU authorized representative is:
Springer Nature Customer Service Center GmbH
Europaplatz 3, 69115 Heidelberg, Germany

Printed by Libri Plureos GmbH
in Hamburg, Germany